Atlas of Airway Surgery

Angelo Ghidini • Francesco Mattioli
Sergio Bottero • Livio Presutti
Editors

Atlas of Airway Surgery

A Step-by-Step Guide Using an Animal Model

Springer

Editors
Angelo Ghidini
University Hospital of Modena
Modena
Italy

Francesco Mattioli
Head and Neck Department
University Hospital of Modena
Modena
Italy

Sergio Bottero
Ped. ENT Dept., Bambino Gesù Hospital
Rome
Italy

Livio Presutti
ENT Department
University of Modena ENT Department
Modena
Italy

ISBN 978-3-319-84229-5 ISBN 978-3-319-49739-6 (eBook)
DOI 10.1007/978-3-319-49739-6

Softcover reprint of the hardcover 1st edition 2017

Printed on acid-free paper

This Springer imprint is published by Springer Nature
The registered company is Springer International Publishing AG
The registered company address is: Gewerbestrasse 11, 6330 Cham, Switzerland

Foreword

It gives me great pleasure to foreword this very unique atlas covering airway reclaiming surgeries. Managing a compromised airway is difficult and requires accurate diagnosis, and meticulous execution of the planned endoscopic and/or surgical interventions. Open techniques are delicate and require adequate training and typically have long learning curves. Mastering of these interventions is best done on animal models and simulating each of the surgical steps. *More you do – better you get* and hence, it is indeed very interesting to try sharpening the surgical skills on animal models as many times before using them in our patients.

The authors have done a commendable job in presenting the anatomy of their animal model, its preparation before the simulation exercises and have given an elaborate description of the various airway surgeries. Every chapter has several illustrations which didactically explain each and every surgical step involved. This atlas is useful to the novice and experienced airway surgeon, and also to all the members of a dedicated airway team responsible in the management of such critically ill patients. It indeed is a *must-have* to all those wanting to start these very difficult interventions – especially when the best chance for the patient lies in the first intervention.

Dr. Kishore Sandu
Chief of Pediatric and Adult Airway Surgical Unit
Department of Otolaryngology and Head – Neck Surgery
Lausanne University Hospital, Lausanne, Switzerland

Contents

1 Anatomy of Animal Model and Comparison to Human

M. Ghirelli, M. Fermi, E. Aggazzotti Cavazza, A. Ghidini, S. Bottero, and L. Presutti

A good knowledge of the anatomical structures of the sheep model is mandatory to perform a good dissection.

In this chapter the anatomical landmarks of the neck and the larynx, internally and externally, are described and compared to the human.

To simplify the organization of the anatomical structures in the sheep's neck, we can divide it into two compartments: the anterior compartment and the posterior compartment.

The anterior compartment includes many noble structures such as vessels, nerves, and glands. It also includes the larynx and the trachea.

The posterior compartment includes mainly paravertebral muscles and the cervical spine (Fig. 1.1).

Similarly the human larynx has the function of air passage, phonation, and sphincter. It extends from the tongue to the trachea.

The ipopharynx is located posterior to the larynx and continues into the esophagus; the prevertebral muscles divides anterior and posterior compartements of the neck.

The larynx is covered superficially by infrahyoid muscles from the cervical bands and skin.

Before starting with neck dissection, it is useful to identify skin landmark of larynx framework (Fig. 1.2).

After skin incision there is a subcutaneous tissue composed of skin subcutaneous tissue and cutaneous colli muscle which is similar to platysma muscle (Fig. 1.3).

The superficial cervical fascia (Fig. 1.2) is quite thicker than the human one but nevertheless is easily dissected with a scalpel or a pair of scissors in order to expose the mid cervical fascia.

The mid cervical fascia is thinner than the superficial one and surrounds the larynx and the infrahyoid compartment (Fig. 1.3).

By opening up the mid cervical fascia, we can approach the infrahyoid region which contains the infrahyoid muscles and the larynx framework (Fig. 1.4).

The larynx is surrounded laterally by the great vessels, sternomastoid muscle and the submandibular glands (Figs. 1.5, 1.6, and 1.7).

Caudal laryngeal nerve in the sheep is similar to recurrent laryngeal nerve (*RLN*) of human. To simplify the explanation, caudal laryngeal nerve is called RLN.

RLNs lie into tracheoesophageal groove (Fig. 1.8) and pass behind the thyroid gland (*TG*) before getting into the larynx through the cricothyroid membrane (Fig. 1.9). Its direction is comparable to the one in the human specimen.

M. Ghirelli (✉) • M. Fermi • E. Aggazzotti Cavazza
A. Ghidini • L. Presutti
Head and Neck Department, University Hospital of Modena, Modena, Italy
e-mail: michael.ghirelli@gmail.com

S. Bottero
Airway Surgery Unit, Laryngotracheal Team Director, Bambino Gesù Children's Hospital, Rome, Italy

A. Ghidini et al. (eds.), *Atlas of Airway Surgery*, DOI 10.1007/978-3-319-49739-6_1

The laryngeal framework is covered by the infrahyoid muscles. Differently from the human, in the sheep these muscles are not fused in the midline (Figs. 1.10a, b, 1.11a and b).

By dissecting the infrahyoid muscles, it is possible to entirely expose the laryngeal framework. The thyrohyoid ligament connects the medial aspect of the thyroid cartilage to the hyoid bone, while the thyrohyoid membrane is more lateral (Fig. 1.12).

Hyoid bone is composed of a body (*B*), a great horn (*GH*), and a lesser horn (*LH*) which is more prominent and articulates with the styloid bone (*SB*) that is longer than human styloid process (Fig. 1.13).

Dissection of the thyrohyoid ligament and thyrohyoid membrane allows the mobilization of the hyoid bone and the exposure of the pre-epiglottic space (Fig. 1.14).

Dissection of the pre-epiglottic space soft tissue allows to get into the ipopharynx (Fig. 1.15).

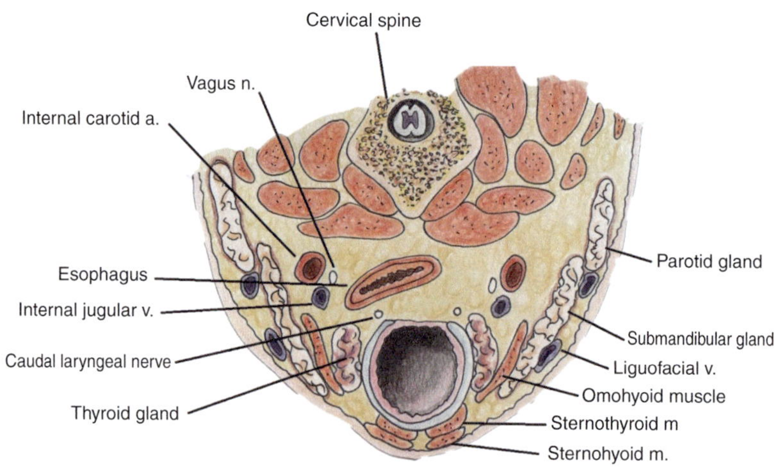

Fig. 1.1 Transverse section of sheep neck. Clearly evidence of anterior and posterior compartments

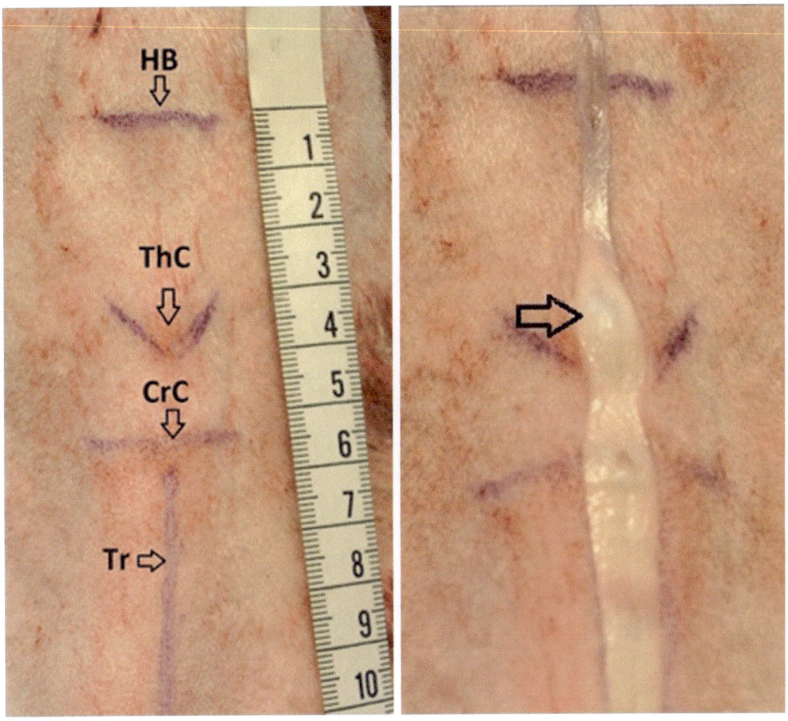

Fig. 1.2 Skin landmarks are hyoid bone (*HB*), thyroid cartilage (*ThC*), cricoid cartilage (*CrC*), and trachea (*Tr*). Superficial cervical fascia (*arrow*)

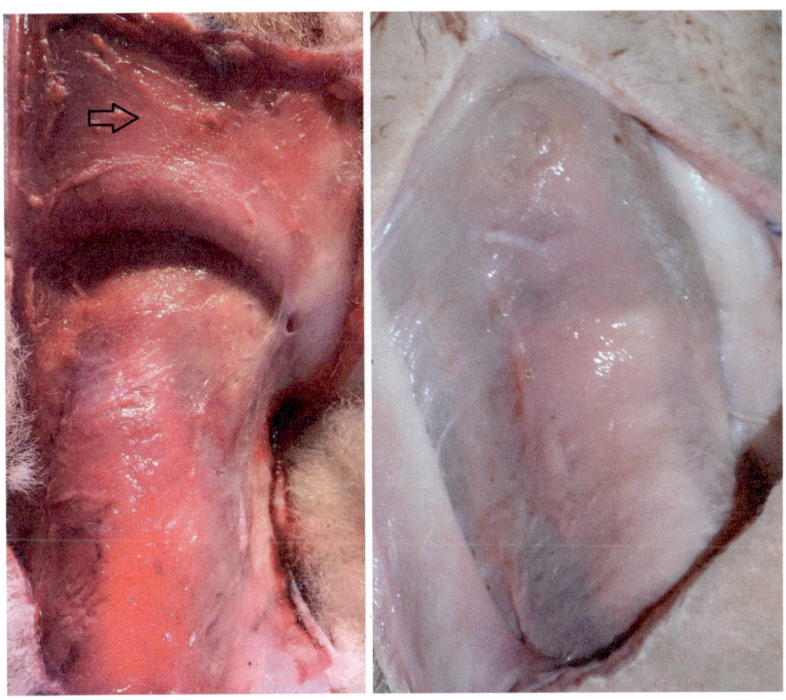

Fig. 1.3 Evidence of mid cervical fascia. The arrow underlines the cutaneous colli muscle included into the superficial flap (*arrow*)

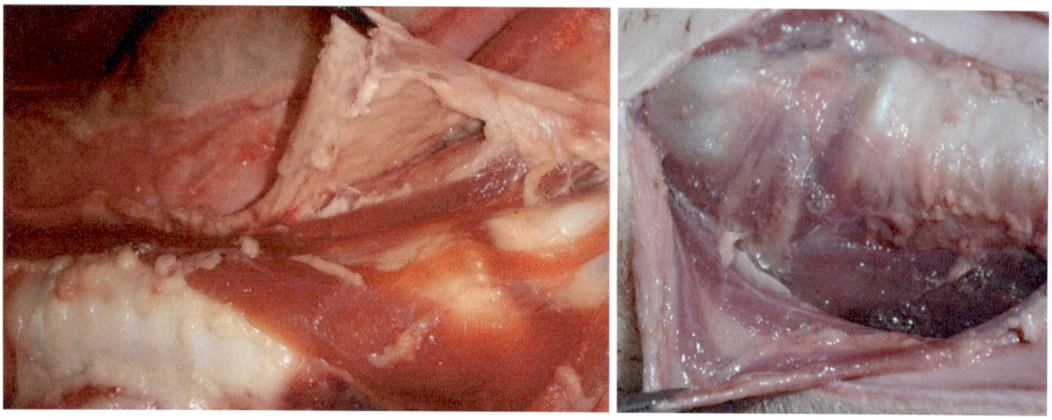

Fig. 1.4 Dissection of mid cervical fascia

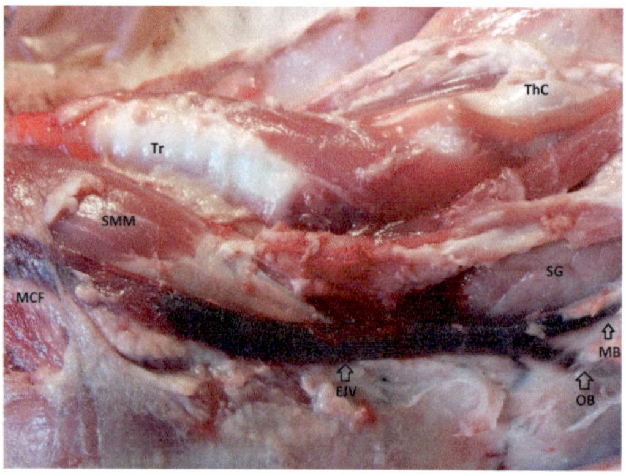

Fig. 1.5 Lateral view. On the midline evidence of larynx in particular thyroid cartilage (*ThC*) and trachea (*Tr*). The mid cervical fascia (*MCF*) was dissected on the midline and preserved at the inferior part in order to show how it surrounds neck structures. Lateral to the larynx evidence of sternomastoid muscle (*SMM*), external jugular vein (*EJV*), and its branches: maxillary (*MB*) and occipital (*OB*). Submandibular gland (*SG*) is also visible in relationship with the maxillary branch of the external jugular vein

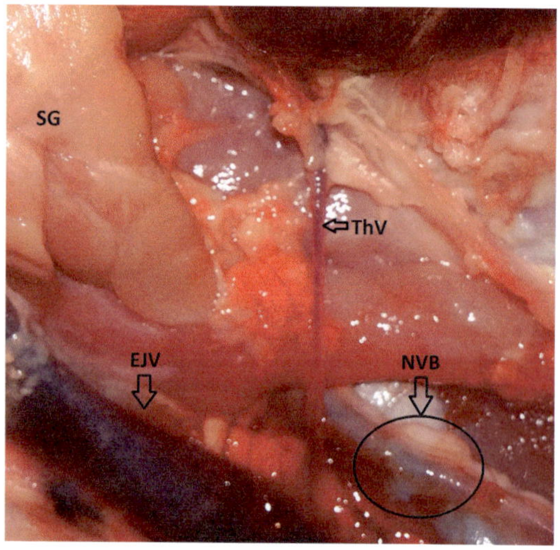

Fig. 1.6 Evidence of the neurovascular bundle (*NVB*) formed by carotid artery, internal jugular vein, and vagus nerve. The external jugular vein (*EJV*) and submandibular gland (*SG*) are located more superficially and laterally. Thyroid vein (*ThV*) arises from jugular vein and reaches the thyroid gland

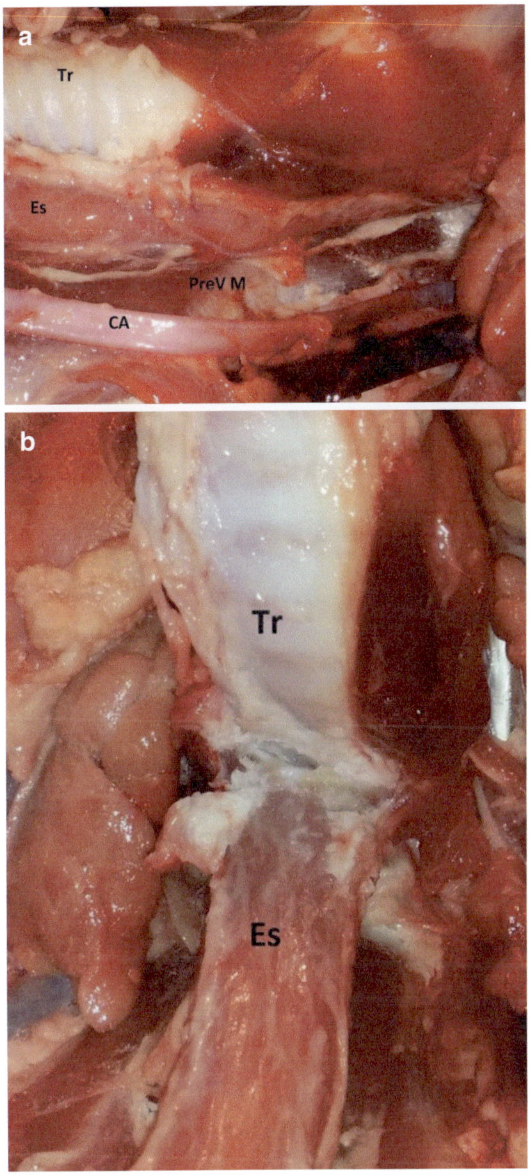

Fig. 1.7 (**a**) Evidence of prevertebral muscles (*PreV M*) on posterior plane. The esophagus (*Es*) lies on the posterior wall of the larynx and trachea (*Tr*). Carotid artery (*CA*) is located laterally to the larynx (**b**) Trachea (*Tr*) was dissected from esophagous (*Es*)

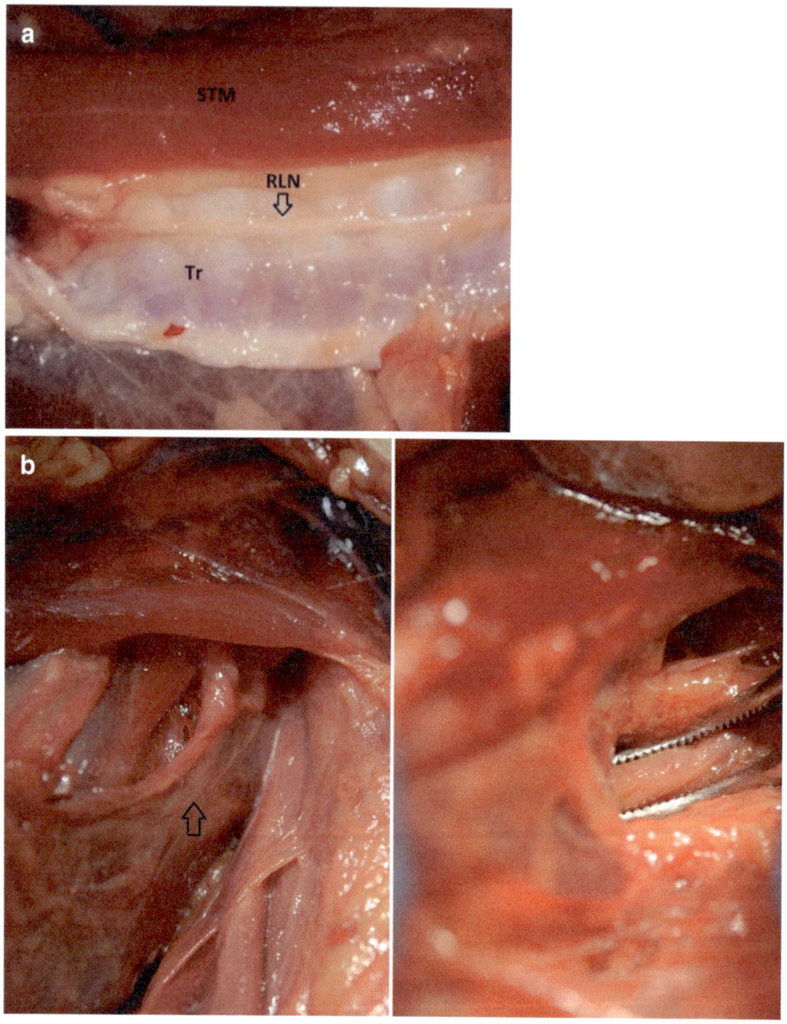

Fig. 1.8 (**a**) *RLN* runs into the tracheoesophageal groove. The nerve lies between the trachea (*Tr*) and the esophagus (*Es*). (**b**) RLN course in human dissection. RLN is covered by fascia (*arrow*). Fascial layer has been dissected showing RLN immediately below

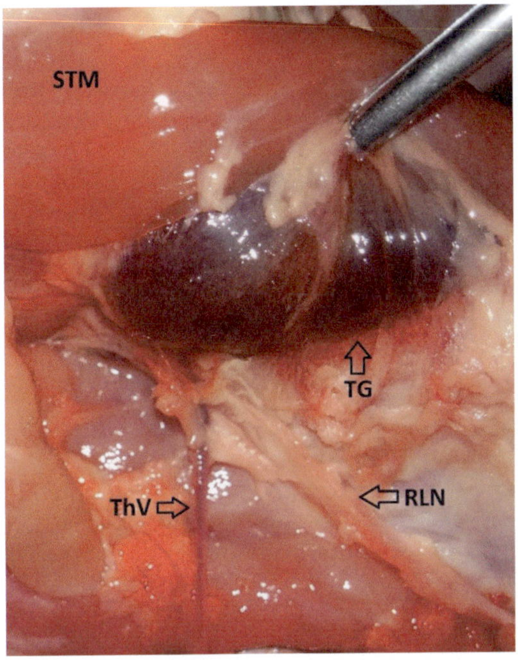

Fig. 1.9 RLN passes behind the thyroid gland (*TG*). Evidence of the thyroid vein (*ThV*) going toward the inferior pole of the thyroid gland

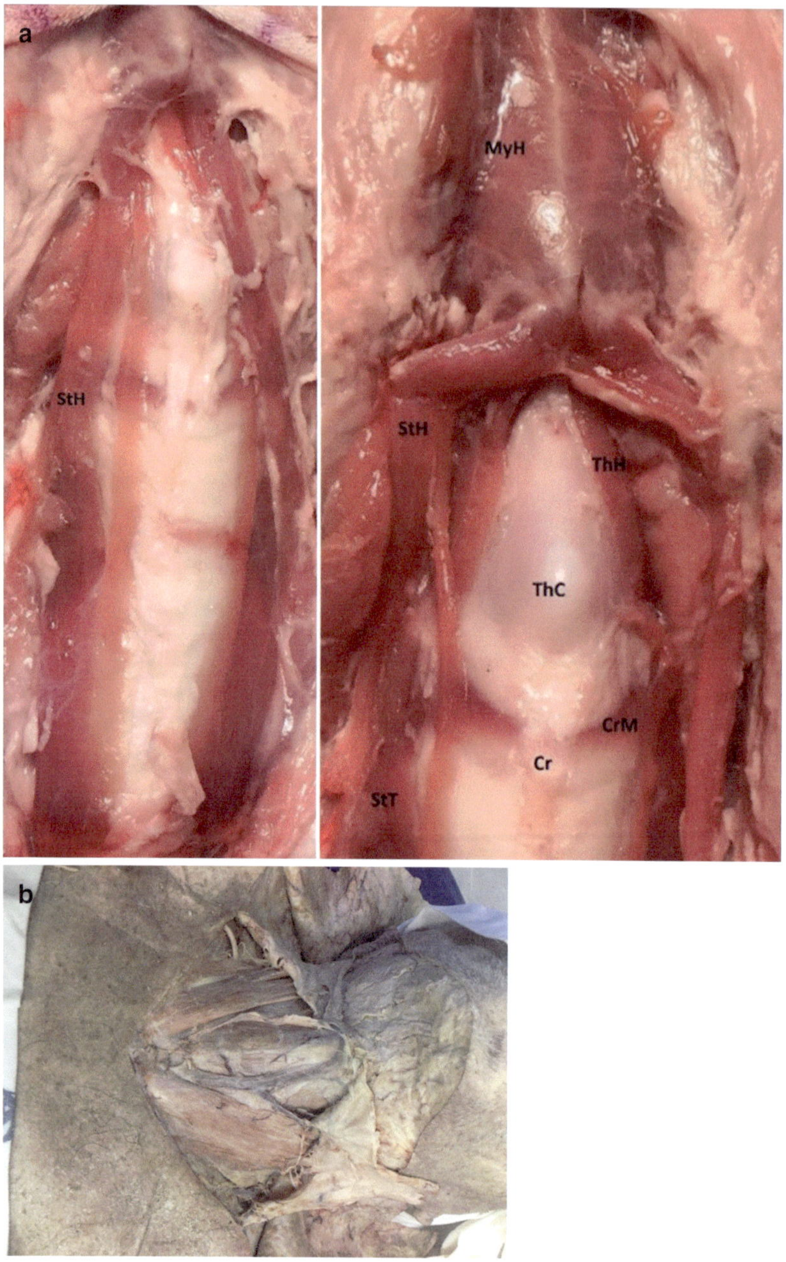

Fig. 1.10 (**a**) Infrahyoid muscles: (*StH*) sternohyoid muscle, (*ThH*) thyrohyoid muscle, and (*StT*) sternothyroid muscle. (*ThC*) thyroid cartilage, (*Cr*) cricoid cartilage, (*CrT*) cricothyroid muscle. In the suprahyoid region, there is the (*MyH*) mylohyoid muscle. (**b**) Infrahyoid muscles in human anatomy

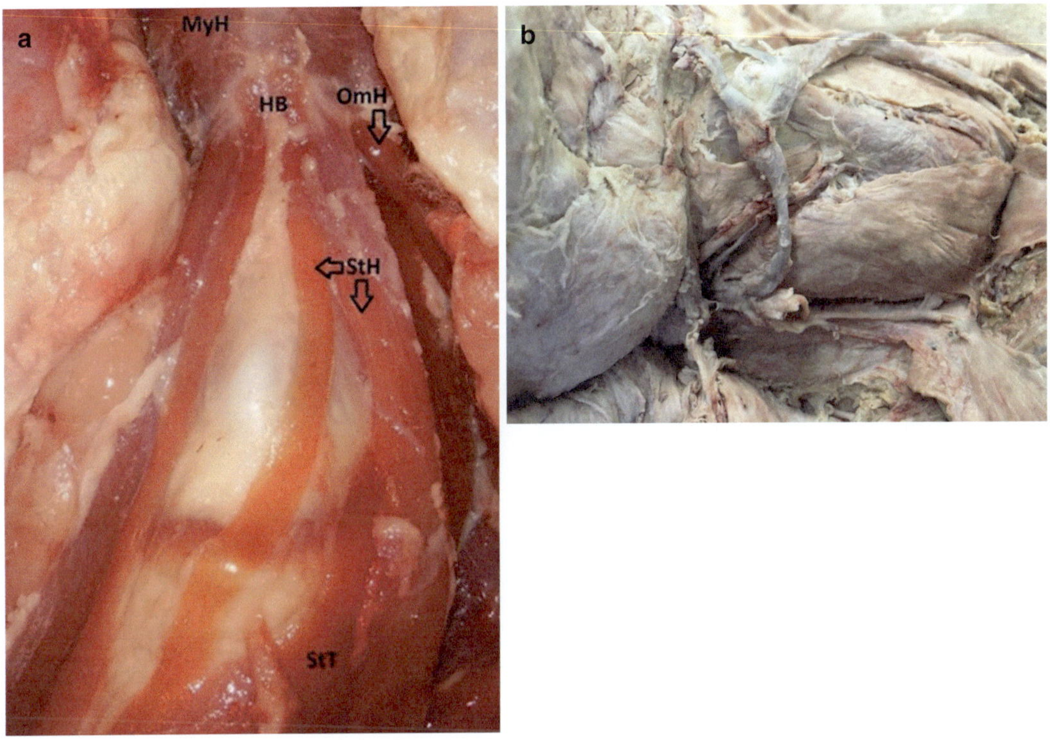

Fig. 1.11 (**a**) Prominence of hyoid bone (*HB*) divides the (*MyH*) mylohyoid muscle from infrahyoid muscles: (*StH*) sternohyoid muscle, (*StT*) sternothyroid muscle, and (*OmH*) omohyoid muscle. (**b**) Lateral view of infrahyoid muscles in human anatomy

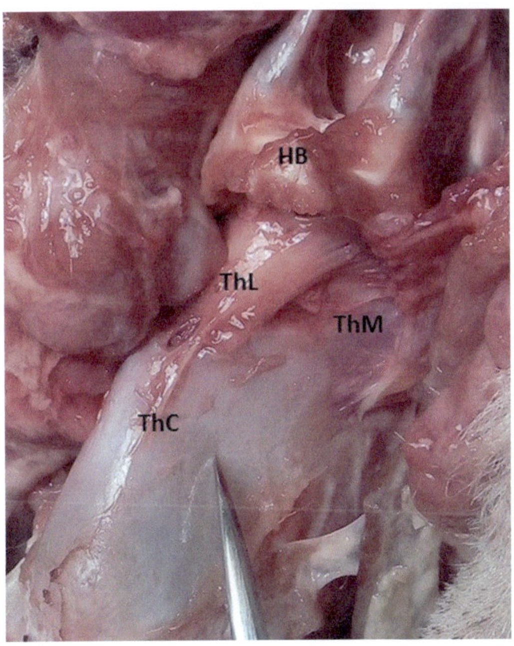

Fig. 1.12 Hyoid bone (*HB*) and thyroid cartilage (*ThC*) connected to the thyrohyoid ligament (*ThL*) and thyrohyoid membrane (*ThM*)

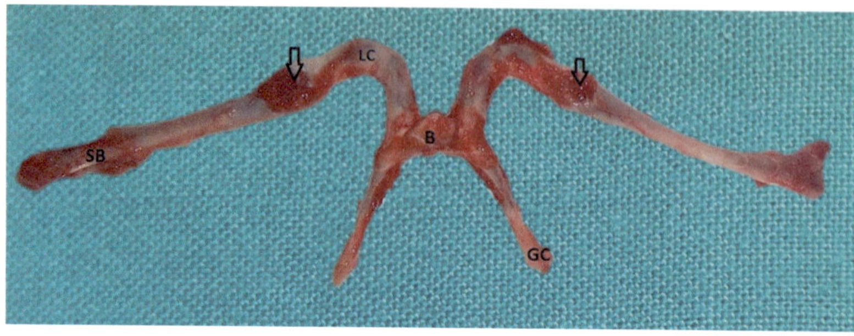

Fig. 1.13 Hyoid bone: body (*B*), greater horn (*GH*), and lesser horn (*LH*). *Black arrow*: articulation between styloid bone (*SB*) and *LH*

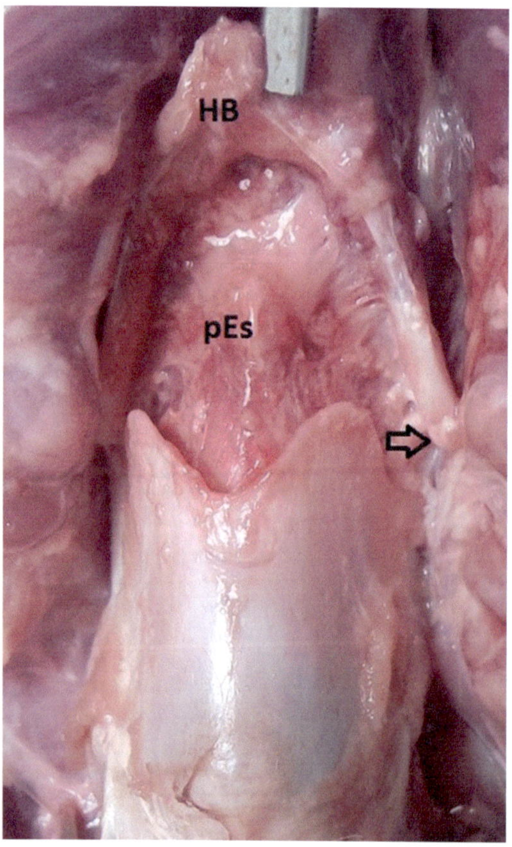

Fig. 1.14 Evidence of tissue located in pre-epiglottic space (*pEs*). Articulation between hyoid bone (*HB*) and thyroid cartilage (*black arrow*)

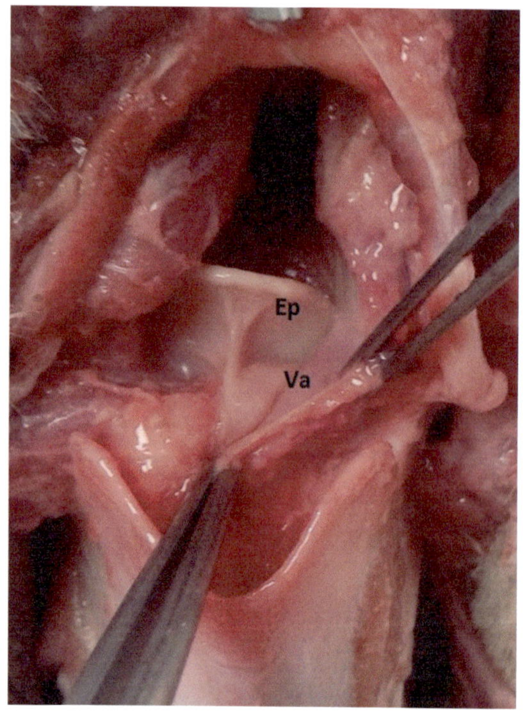

Fig. 1.15 pEs dissected, evidence of vallecula and epiglottis and posterior pharynx wall

1.1 Laryngeal Framework

The larynx framework is formed by a series of cartilages interconnected by ligaments and fibrous membranes and moved by a number of muscles.

To resume, the laryngeal cartilages are the thyroid cartilage, the cricoid cartilage, the epiglottis, and the two arytenoid cartilages.

1.1.1 Thyroid Cartilage

The thyroid cartilage in the largest cartilage of the laryngeal skeleton. It consists of two quadrilateral lamina fused on the midline. Superiorly the laminae are separated by a V-shaped incisure, the superior thyroid notch (Fig. 1.16).

Inferiorly, the thyroid cartilage is connected to the cricoid cartilage thanks to cricothyroid ligament which attaches on the inferior thyroid notch. The cricothyroid membrane connects the inferior border of thyroid cartilage with superior border of cricoid cartilage (Fig. 1.17).

The angle between the thyroid laminae is smaller than the human one (89° vs 54°), while the laryngeal height is significantly greater.

The oblique line, when infrahyoid muscles are still attached, is located at the inferior border of the thyroid cartilage. This anatomical feature determines that infrahyoid muscles do not make union at the midline like in the human [1].

The posterior border is thick and rounded and receives fibers from pharyngeal constrictor muscles. On its upper part, the superior horn is connected with the hyoid bone by means of the thyrohyoid ligament. The inferior horn is short and thick. It is connected with the posterior part of cricoid cartilage forming the cricothyroid joint (Fig. 1.18).

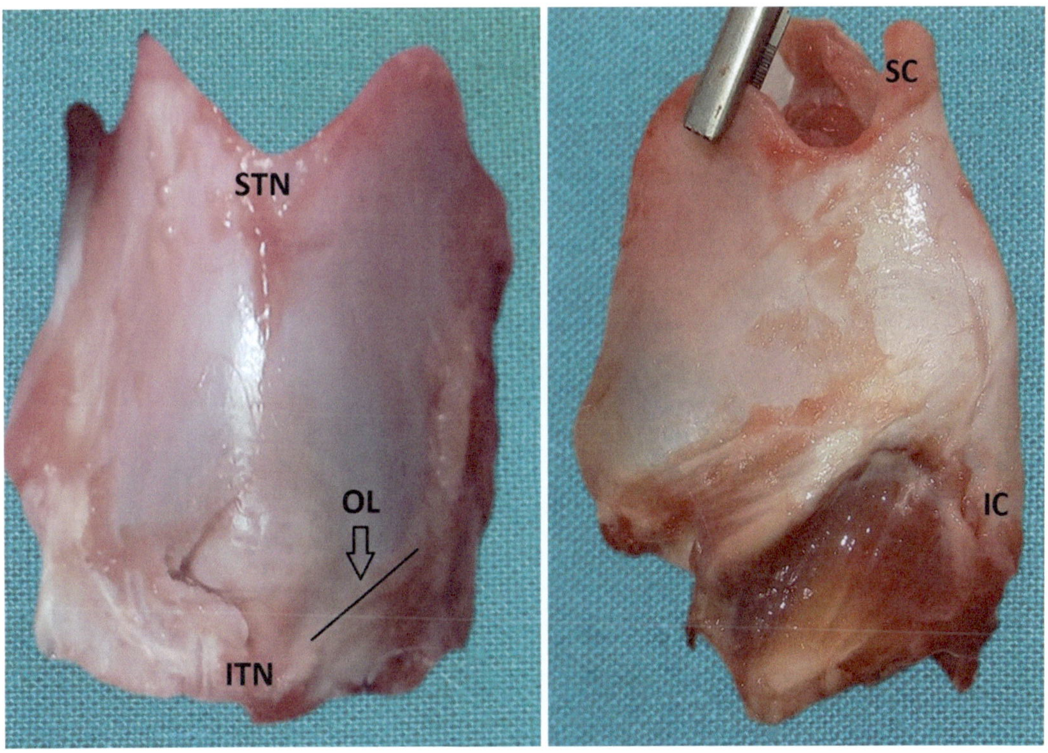

Fig. 1.16 Thyroid cartilage on frontal and sagittal view. Superior thyroid notch (*STN*) and inferior thyroid notch (*ITN*). Oblique line on the inferior part of cartilage (*OL*). Superior horn (*SH*) and inferior horn (*IH*) articulated with cricoid cartilage

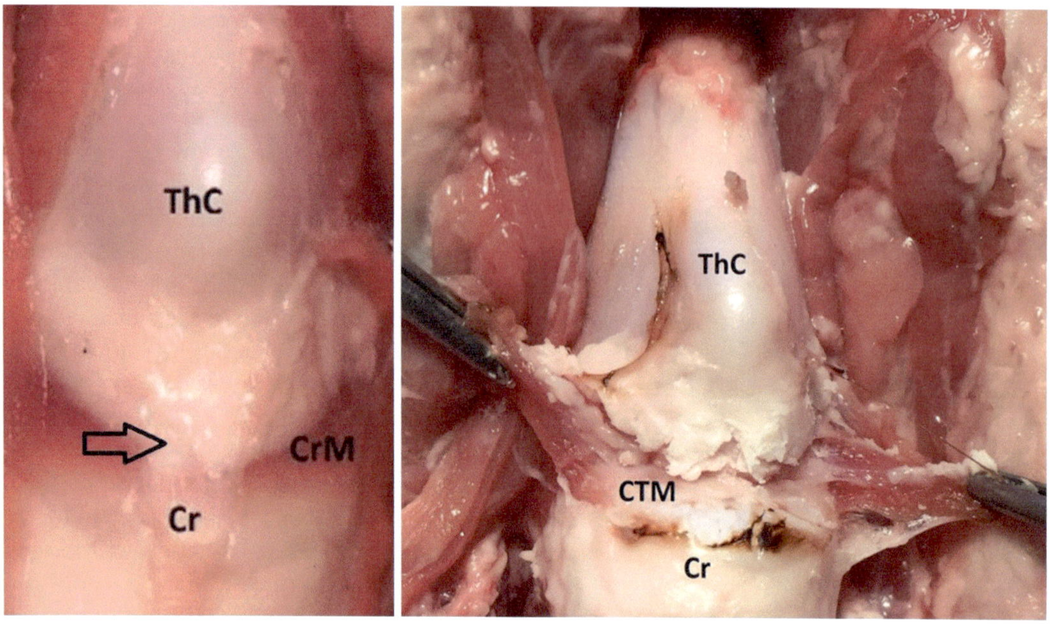

Fig. 1.17 Connection between cricoid (*Cr*) and thyroid cartilage (*ThC*). The *arrow* shows the cricothyroid ligament. The cricothyroid membrane (*CTM*) is exposed by dissecting the cricothyroid muscles (*CrM*)

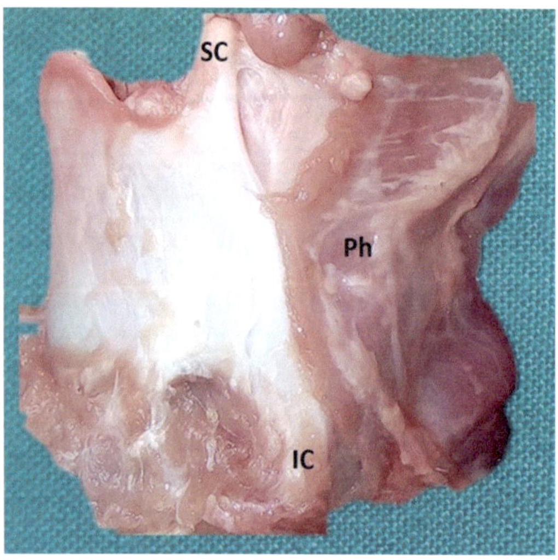

Fig. 1.18 Pharynx constrictor muscles (*Ph*) attached on the posterior border of thyroid cartilage

1.1.2 Cricoid Cartilage

The ovine cricoid cartilage is similar to the human one. The articular facet of arytenoid cartilage is significantly larger because sheep arytenoid cartilage is bigger than human one. Cricoid arch is concave and thinner than in humans.

Posterior view of larynx shows great similarities with the human one. The main difference results in arytenoids conformation (Fig. 1.19).

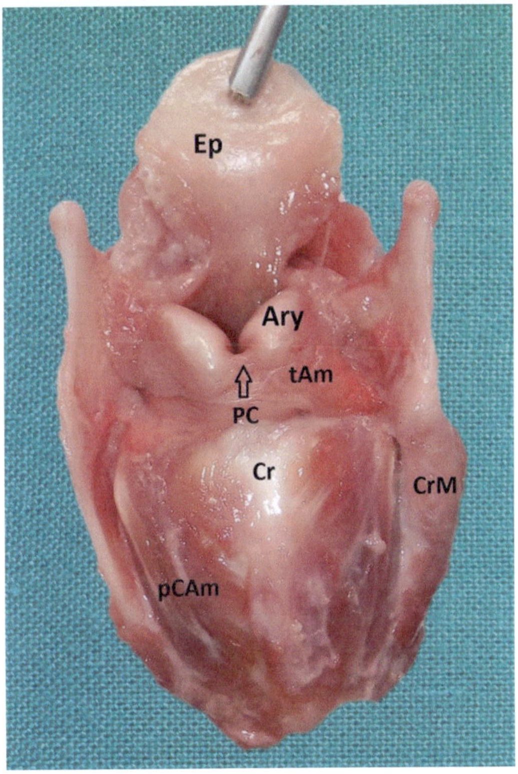

Fig. 1.19 Epiglottis (*Ep*) and petioles in the anterior aspect of the larynx. Arytenoids (*Ary*) and transverse arytenoid muscles (*tAm*). Posterior commissure (*PC*) covered by mucosa. Cricoid cartilage (*Cr*) and posterior cricoarytenoid muscles (*pCAm*) and cricothyroid muscles (*CrM*)

1.2 Endolaryngeal Anatomy

Internally the anatomical configuration seems to be similar to the human one (Fig. 1.20).

The main differences from endolaryngeal human anatomy are (Fig. 1.21):

- Very large "comma-shaped/hockey-stick" arytenoids
- Absence of Morgagni's ventricle (true vocal folds are clearly recognizable)
- Reduced interarytenoid space
- Thinner interarytenoid muscle

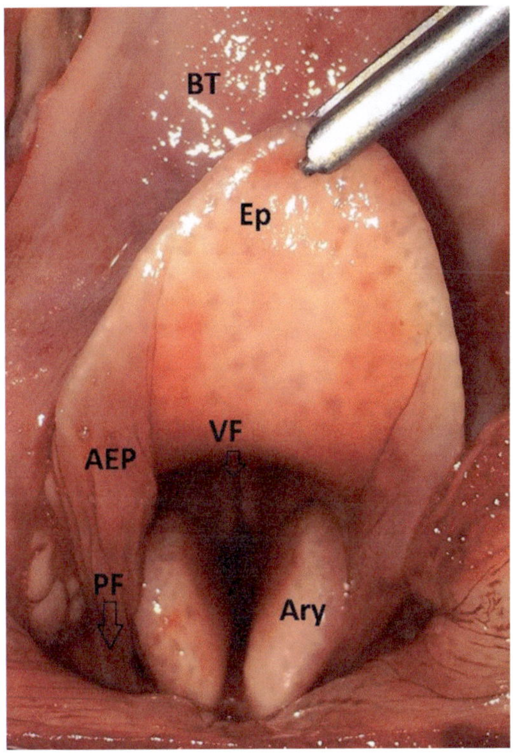

Fig. 1.20 Base of tongue (*BT*). Epiglottis (*Ep*), aryepiglottic fold (*AEP*), piriform fossa (*PF*). Vocal fold (*VF*)

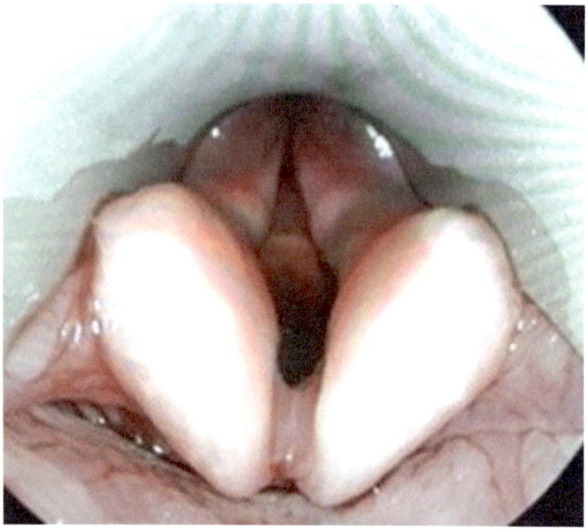

Fig. 1.21 Endoscopic view of the glottis plane

1.2.1 Coronal View of Endolaryngeal Anatomy (Fig. 1.22)

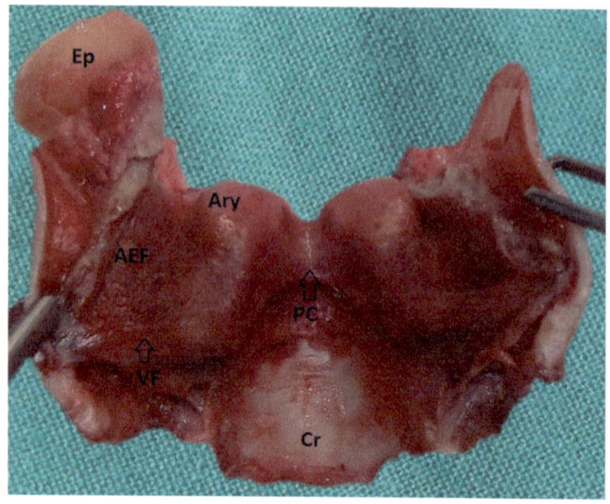

Fig. 1.22 Larynx split on the midline. Evidence of posterior part of cricoid cartilage (*Cr*). Arytenoids (*Ary*) articulated on cricoid cartilage and their union at posterior commissure (*PC*). Vocal fold goes from anterior commissure to arytenoid cartilages. Superiorly there are aryepiglottic folds (*AEP*) and epiglottis (*Ep*)

1.2.2 Sagittal View of Endolaryngeal Anatomy (Fig. 1.23)

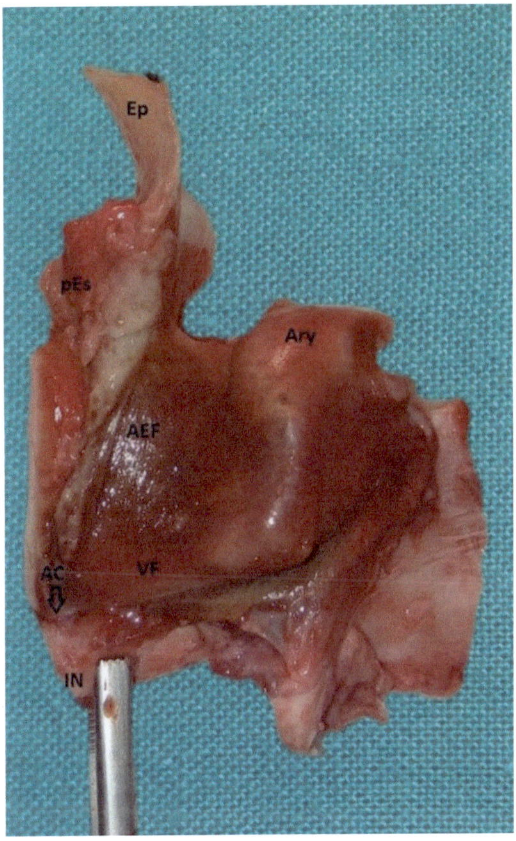

Fig. 1.23 Anterior commissure (*AC*) is located on the midline 10 mm above inferior notch of thyroid cartilage (*IN*). Evidence of arytenoid (*Ary*), vocal fold (*VF*), and aryepiglottic fold (*AEF*). The pre-epiglottis space (*pEs*) is placed anterior to the epiglottis (*Ep*)

Reference

1. Hunter EJ, Titze IR (2005) Individual subject laryngeal dimensions of multiple mammalian species for biomechanical models. Ann Otol Rhinol Laryngol 114(10):809–818

How to Prepare an Animal Model

2

M. Bettini, M. Menichetti, M.P. Alberici, E. Aggazzotti Cavazza, A. Ghidini, A. Camurri, F. Mattioli, and L. Presutti

Core Messages

The standard method for teaching airways surgery is human cadaver head and neck dissections, but supplying human body cadavers is very difficult. Sheep neck has great similarities with humans in size of the organs so it represents a cheap and practical model which can be used to learn airways surgery.

2.1 Introduction

With respect to ethical issues and practice, an attempt for live operation should not be considered as the ideal place to learn airways surgery. This surgery can lead to many complications and it has high morbidity and mortality.

The standard method for teaching airways surgery is human cadaver head and neck dissections. However, in many countries, supplying human body cadavers is very difficult.

Performing airways surgery on an animal model is very useful to learn different surgical approaches and operative techniques. Moreover the preclinical studies on animal models are necessary for the development of new techniques in airways surgery.

Currently many large animal models like sheep are used for surgical training [1, 2], so as goats [3], monkeys [4, 5], and pigs [6].

Sheep cadaver is a cost-effective and useful model for the first step of the learning curve [7]. They have been employed for many years in the orthopedic, neurosurgical [8], and ENT researches [9].

Sheep neck has great similarities with humans in size of the organs so it represents a cheap and practical model which can be used to learn airways surgery.

M. Bettini (✉) • M. Menichetti • M.P. Alberici
E. Aggazzotti Cavazza • A. Ghidini • F. Mattioli
L. Presutti
Head and Neck Department, University Hospital of Modena, Modena, Italy
e-mail: margherita.bettini86@gmail.com

A. Camurri
Veterinary Assistant of University of Modena, Modena, Italy

A. Ghidini et al. (eds.), *Atlas of Airway Surgery*, DOI 10.1007/978-3-319-49739-6_2

2.2 Instrumentation and Equipment

If possible it is better to work in pairs.

Before starting your laboratory session, you should have these materials on hand (Fig. 2.1):

- Dissection tray or a diaper
- Dissection tools: scalpel N°15 and 11 (Fig. 2.2); needle driver (Fig. 2.3); surgical and anatomic forceps (Fig. 2.4); small curved mosquito forceps (Fig. 2.5); Kocher's forceps (Fig. 2.6); Mayo, curved, and straight iris scissors (Fig. 2.7); suture threads 1,0, 2–0, 3–0, 4–0 (Fig. 2.8); Killian's speculum (Fig. 2.9); small retractors (Fig. 2.10); and a suction cannula (Fig. 2.11)
- Medical gauzes
- Paper towel
- A sheep head including the neck (see paragraph below)
- Our atlas

Set up the diaper on the bench and then the dissection tray on the diaper. Obtain dissection instruments and finally put the head into the dissection tray or on the diaper with the neck extended in the dorsal recumbent position (Fig. 2.12).

Remember to practice safe hygiene when dissecting: do not place your hands near your mouth or eyes while handling specimens; wear lab gloves, lab coat, and goggles.

Although the medical risk of contracting animal diseases is low, precautions need to be taken when using this model. The specimen should be provided from a known source and from animals under official veterinary control. We also recommend that surgical instruments used in the study aren't used on human subjects and all sterilization measures should be absolutely rigorous.

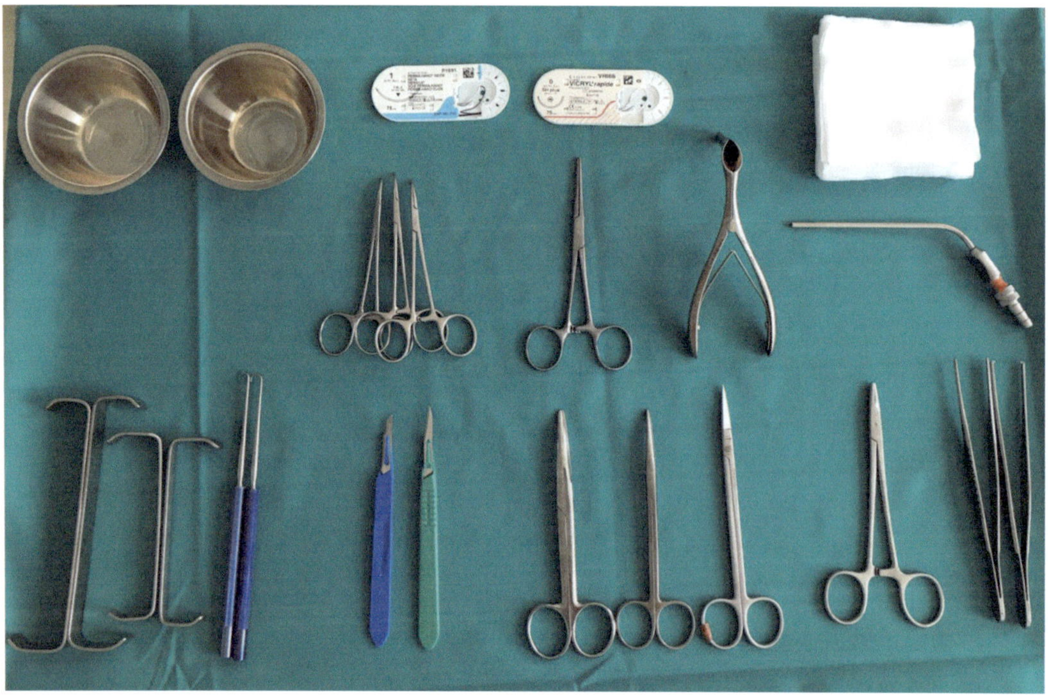

Fig. 2.1 Set of surgical instruments

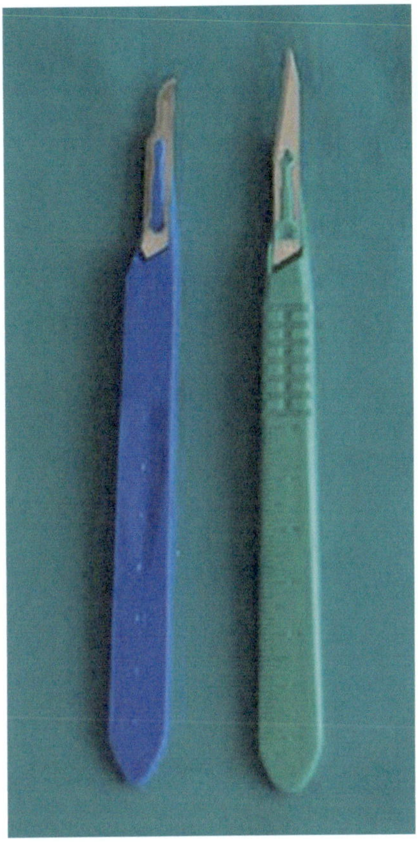

Fig. 2.2 Scalpels

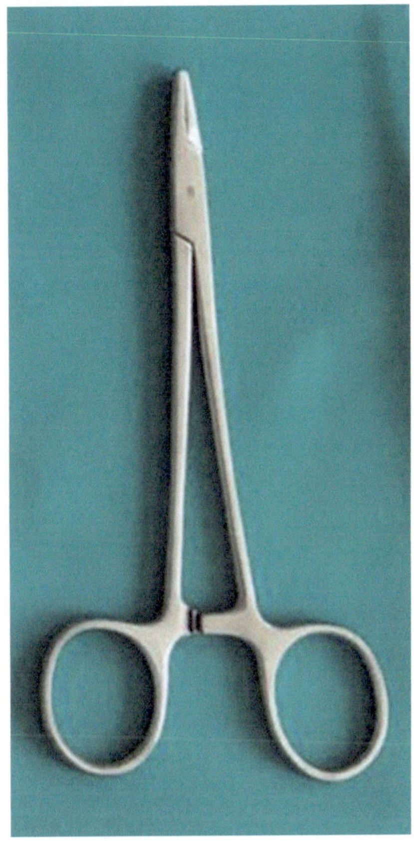

Fig. 2.3 Needle driver

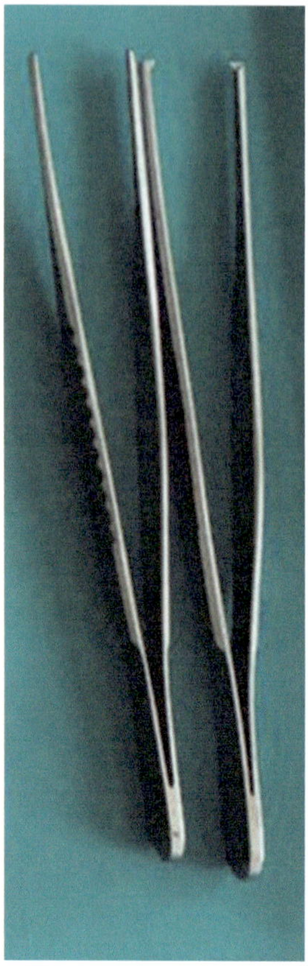

Fig. 2.4 Surgical and anatomic forceps

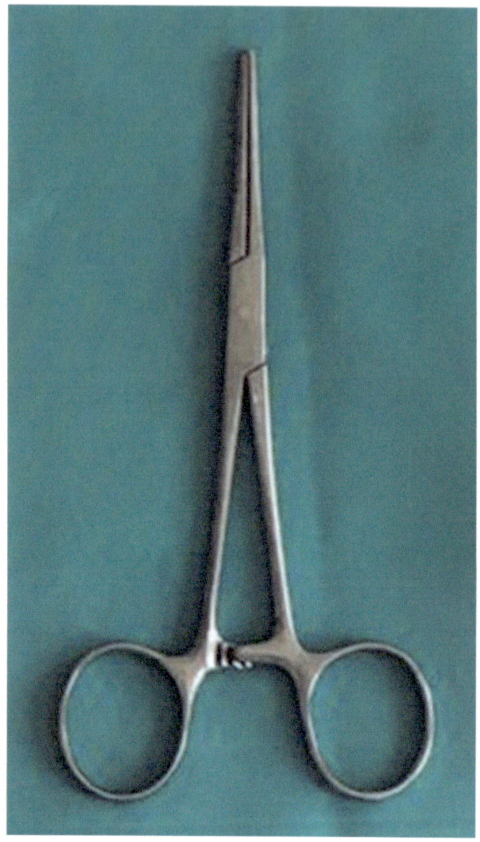

Fig. 2.6 Kocher's forceps

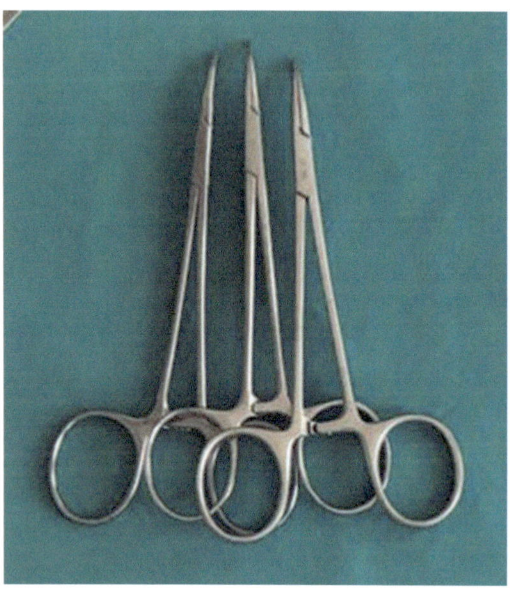

Fig. 2.5 Curved mosquito forceps

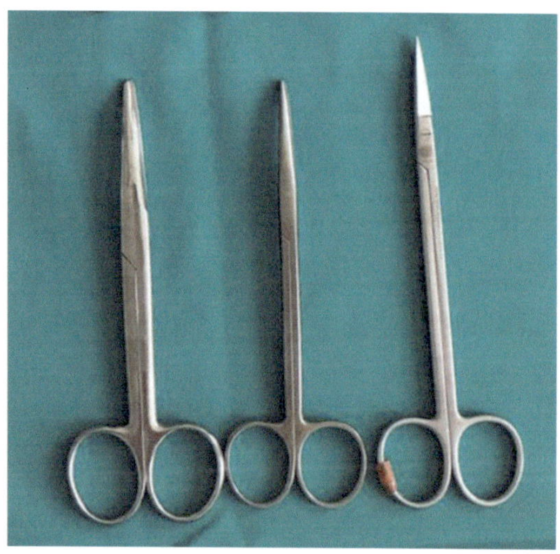

Fig. 2.7 Scissors

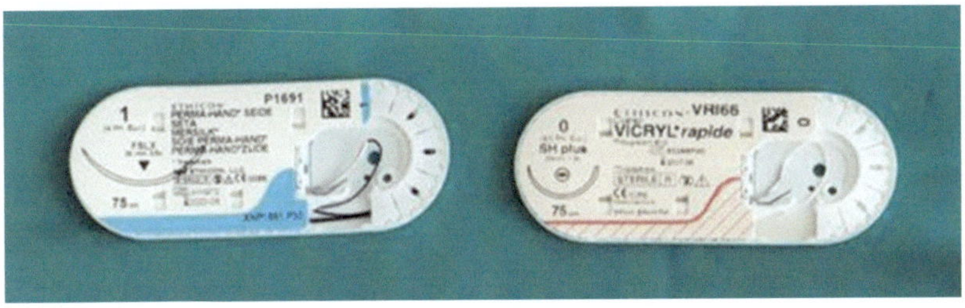

Fig. 2.8 Suture threads

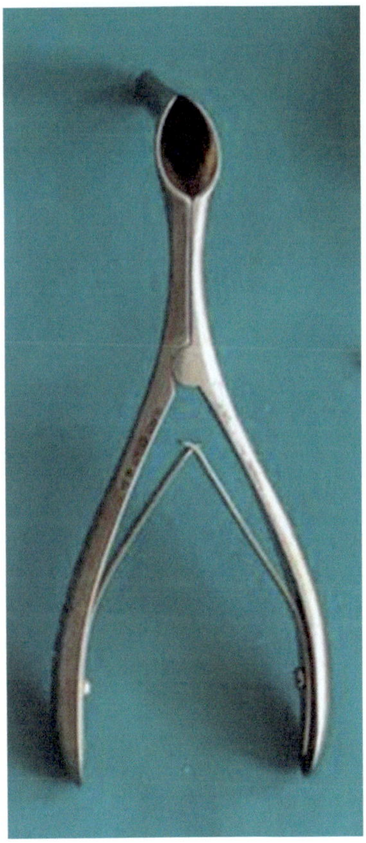

Fig. 2.9 Killian's speculum

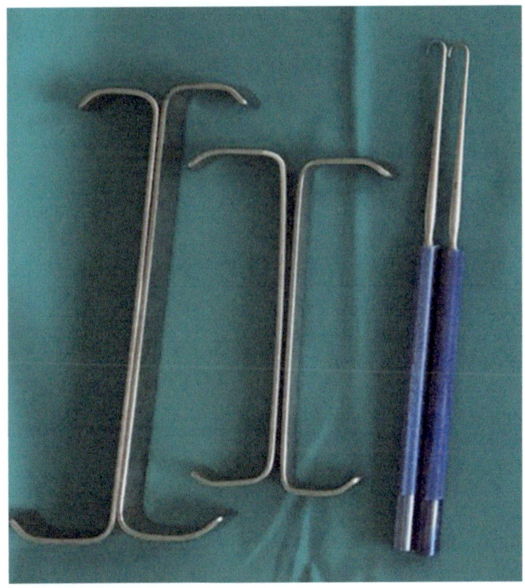

Fig. 2.10 Retractors

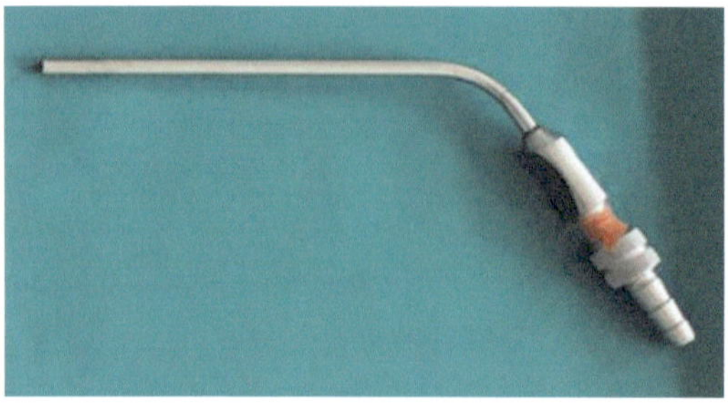

Fig. 2.11 Suction cannula

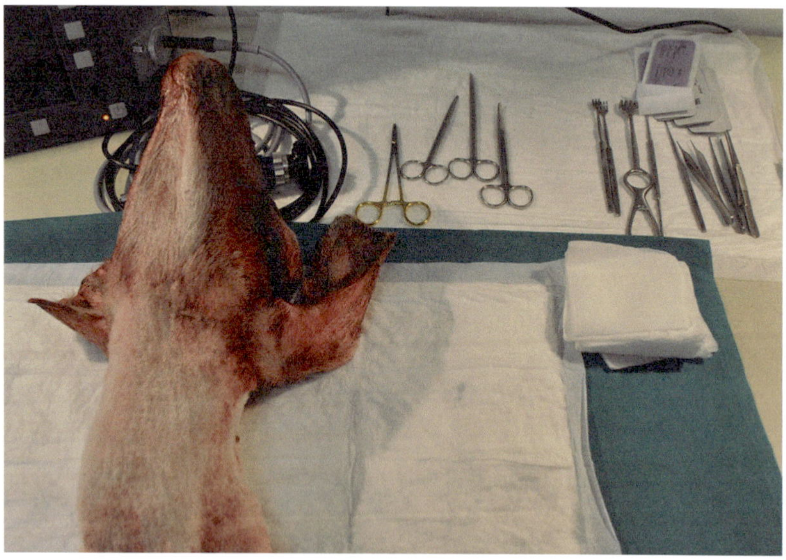

Fig. 2.12 Setup of the surgical field

2.3 Model Preparation

The sheep head is purchased fresh from an abattoir at a low cost. It must include all the cervical region till to the superior edge of the sternum and of the collarbones (Fig. 2.13). We suggest you to use head from adult animal, older about 6 months because the size of the larynx and the trachea is similar to human's one.

The head has been unfrozen for at least 24 h.

An electric razor, a sheep shearing machine, or scissors (Figs. 2.14 and 2.15) are useful to shave the anterior part of the sheep's neck (Fig. 2.16).

When not used, the specimen can be frozen and unfrozen again when necessary.

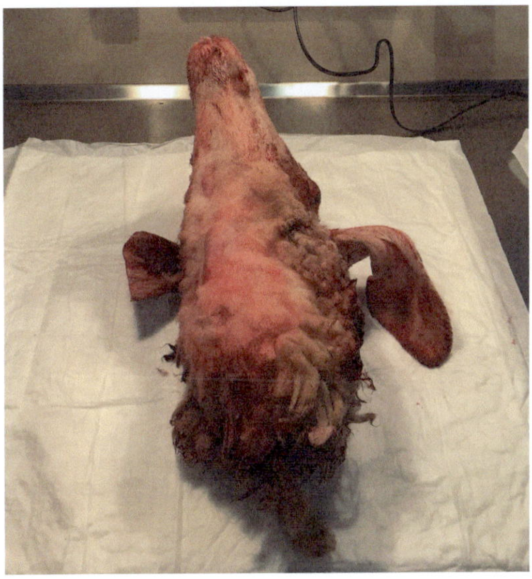

Fig. 2.13 Sheep head including cervical region before shaving

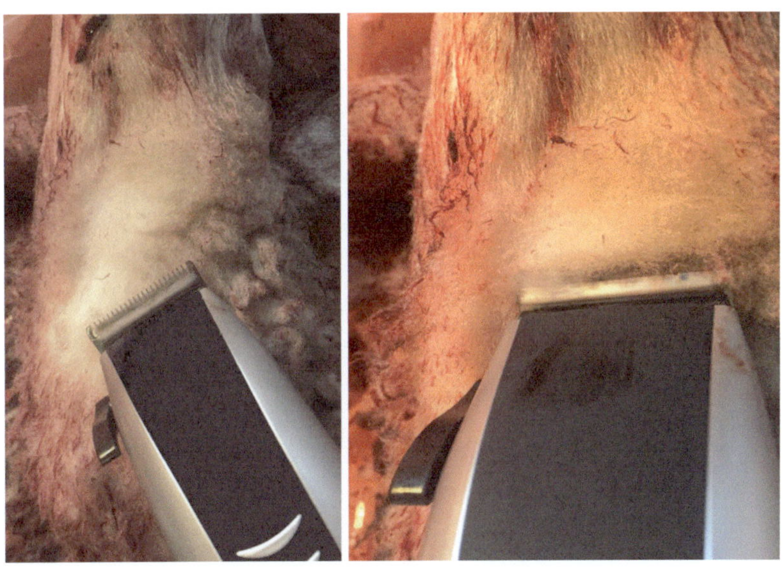

Fig. 2.14 Shaving of the anterior part of the neck lamb with electric razor

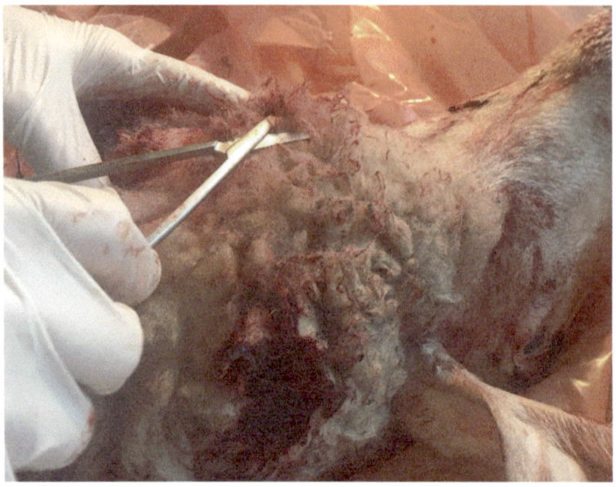

Fig. 2.15 Shaving of the anterior part of the neck lamb with scissors

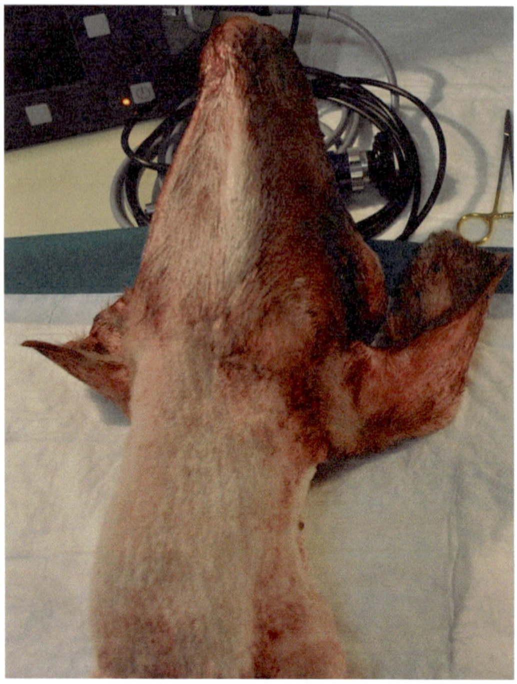

Fig. 2.16 Sheep head after shaving

Take-Home Message

- Performing airways surgery on an animal model is very useful to learn different surgical approaches and operative techniques.
- Sheep cadaver is a cost-effective and useful model for the first step of the learning curve of airway procedures.
- Few instruments are necessary to perform most of all procedures.
- The sheep head needs to be accurately prepared before dissection.

References

1. Brumund KT, Graham SM, Beck KC, Hoffman EA, McLennan G (2004) The effect of maxillary sinus antrostomy size on xenon ventilation in the sheep model. Otolaryngol Head Neck Surg 131(4):528–533
2. Acar B, Gunbey E, Babademez MA, Karabulut H, Gunbey HP, Karasen RM (2010) Utilization and dissection for endoscopic sinus surgery training in the residency program. J Craniofac Surg 21(6):1715–1718
3. Nevins M, Kirker-Head C, Nevins M, Wozney JA, Palmer R, Graham D (1996) Bone formation in the goat maxillary sinus induced by absorbable collagen sponge implants impregnated with recombinant human bone morphogenetic protein-2. Int J Periodontics Restorative Dent 16(1):8–19
4. Kirker-Head CA, Nevins M, Palmer R, Nevins ML, Schelling SH (1997) A new animal model for maxillary sinus floor augmentation: evaluation parameters. Int J Oral Maxillofac Implants 12(3):403–411
5. Estaca E, Cabezas J, Usón J, Sánchez-Margallo F, Morell E, Latorre R (2008) Maxillary sinus-floor elevation: an animal model. Clin Oral Implants Res 19(10):1044–1048
6. Terris DJ, Haus BM, Nettar K, Ciecko S, Gourin CG (2004) Prospective evaluation of endoscopic approaches to the thyroid compartment. Laryngoscope 114(8):1377–1382
7. Potes JC (2008) The sheep as an animal model in orthopaedic research. Experimental Pathology and Health Sciences 2(1):29–32
8. Hamamcioglu MK, Hicdonmez T, Tiryaki M, Cobanoglu S (2008) A laboratory training model in fresh cadaveric sheep brain for microneurosurgical dissection of cranial nerves in posterior fossa. Br J Neurosurg 22(6):769–771
9. Ozdemir NG, Is M, Bozkurt SU, Kilic K, Seker A (2015) Superior medullary velum: anatomical-histological study in the sheep brain and a preliminary tractographic study in the human brain. Turk Neurosurg 25(2):246–251

3 Tracheotomy

M. Menichetti, E. Aggazzotti Cavazza, M.P. Alberici, F. Mattioli, A. Ghidini, S. Bottero, and L. Presutti

Core Messages

- Current indications for tracheotomy include:
  - Laryngotracheal stenosis (LTS)
  - Prolonged ventilatory support
  - Pulmonary toilet for permanent aspiration
- Proper tracheostomy placement:
  - For prolonged ventilatory support or pulmonary toilet:
    Third and fourth tracheal ring
  - For impending LTS:
    First tracheal ring
    Sixth and seventh tracheal ring
  - For tracheal stenosis or recurrent stenosis at the tracheostomy site:
    Through tracheal stenosis
    Through former tracheostoma
  - For distal intrathoracic stenosis:
    Close to thoracic inlet (sixth or seventh tracheal ring), with long cannula to stent the distal stenosis

3.1 Introduction

There are numerous indications for performing a tracheotomy. The oldest remains acute upper airway obstruction, but in more recent times, this surgery has been utilized in the setting of prolonged intubation, inability to extubate, maxillofacial trauma, laryngeal or neck trauma, obstructive sleep apnea, and as an adjunctive treatment in head and neck oncology whether for tumor ablation, secondary effects of radiation therapy, or reconstruction of the maxilla or mandible. Inability to extubate can be due to multiple factors related to pulmonary disease, immobility of the vocal fold, and so on [1–9]. The duration of intubation before a tracheostomy is recommended and varies widely and must be decided on a case-by-case basis, depending on the nature and prognosis of the primary disease, as well as the presence of comorbidities. Severe anterior neck burns, vascular anomalies of the lower neck, and the need for high peak inspiratory pressures that may cause pneumomediastinum/pneumothorax are all contraindications to performing a tracheotomy [10].

M. Menichetti (✉) • E. Aggazzotti Cavazza
M.P. Alberici • F. Mattioli • A. Ghidini • S. Bottero
L. Presutti
Head and Neck Departement, University Hospital of Modena, Modena, Italy
e-mail: marcellamenichetti@hotmail.it

A. Ghidini et al. (eds.), *Atlas of Airway Surgery*, DOI 10.1007/978-3-319-49739-6_3

3.2 Instrumentation and Equipment

If possible it is better to work in pairs.

Before starting your laboratory session, you should have these materials on hand (Fig. 3.1):

- Dissection tray or a diaper
- Dissection tools: scalpel N°15 and 11 (Fig. 3.1a); needle driver (Fig. 3.1b); surgical and anatomic forceps (Fig. 3.1c); small curved mosquito forceps (Fig. 3.1d); Kocher's forceps (Fig. 3.1e); Mayo, curved, and straight iris scissors (Fig. 3.1f); suture threads 1,0, 2–0, 3–0, 4–0 (Fig. 3.1g); Killian's speculum (Fig. 3.1h); small retractors (Fig. 3.1i); and a suction cannula (Fig. 3.1j)
- Medical gauzes (Fig. 3.1k)
- Paper towel

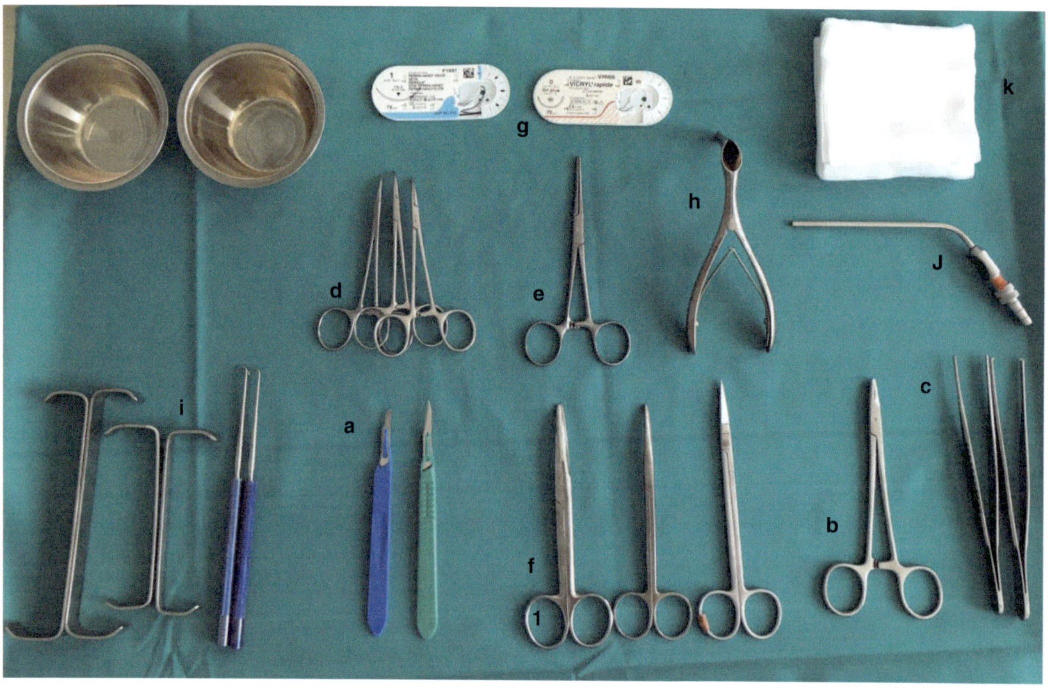

Fig. 3.1 Set of surgical instruments

Step 1 Skin Landmark Identification

Recognizing the main landmarks on the skin (Fig. 3.2) is probably the most simple and fundamental step in all surgical head and neck procedures. Identification by palpation of laryngeal framework in sheep animal model is quite similar to human. Before starting the procedure, it is useful to identify:

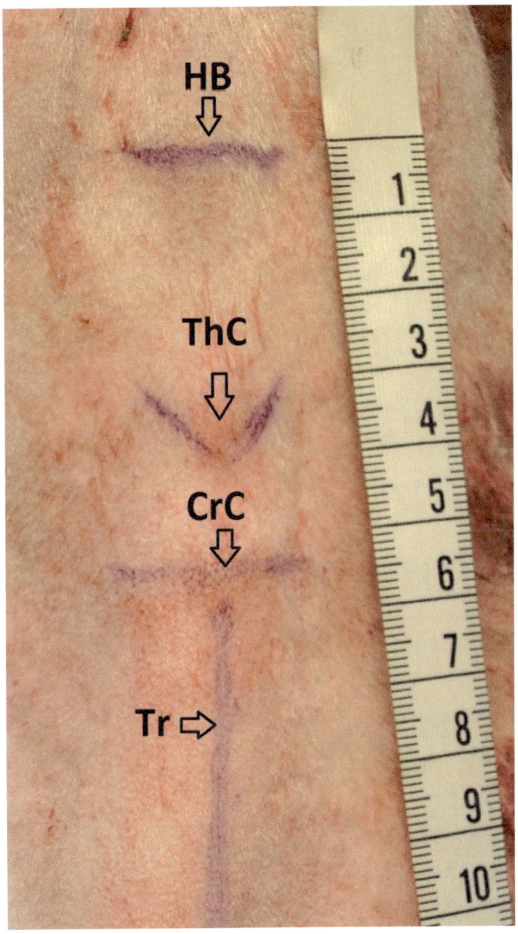

Fig. 3.2 Superficial landmark identification. *HB* hyoid bone, partial cover by the muscles, *ThC* thyroid cartilage, *Cr* cricoid cartilage, *Tr* trachea

Step 2 Superficial Layer Dissection
Make a horizontal incision about 3–4 cm in order to show the superficial fascia that covers the muscles of the neck (Fig. 3.3). Incision could be performed with 10 or 15 blade.

In this step the main goal is to elevate only a cutaneous and subcutaneous flap.

When all superficial fascia is exposed, the surgeon has to dissect it on the midline with surgical scissor or blade (Fig. 3.3).

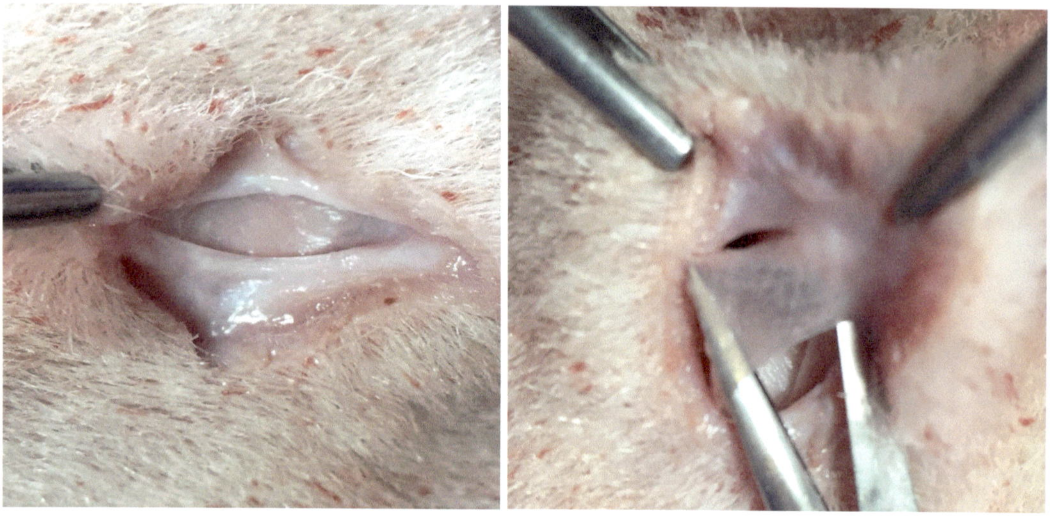

Fig. 3.3 Skin incision; superficial cervical fascia dissected. *Below* structures that are covered by its fascia

Step 3 Laryngeal and Tracheal Framework Identification
When the dissection of the superficial layers is completed, it is important to identify the main structures of laryngeal and tracheal framework and muscles surrounding the larynx (Fig. 3.4).

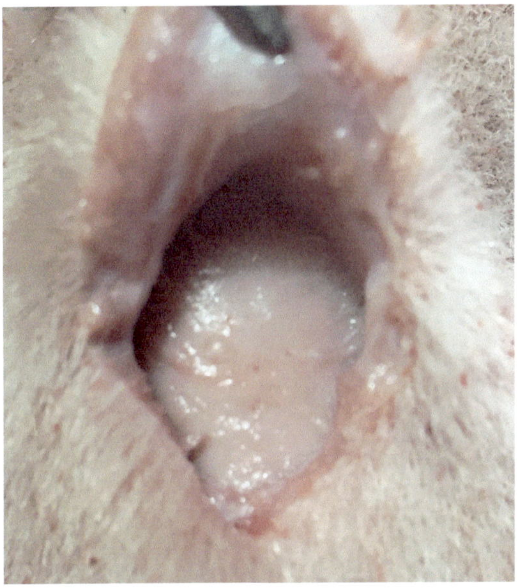

Fig. 3.4 Larynx exposed with muscles surrounding it

Step 4 Infrahyoid Muscle Dissection
This step simulates the strap muscle dissection on the midline performed in the human procedure in order to expose the trachea. Sheep thyroid does not have an isthmus so it is not necessary to split thyroid gland on the midline (Fig. 3.5).

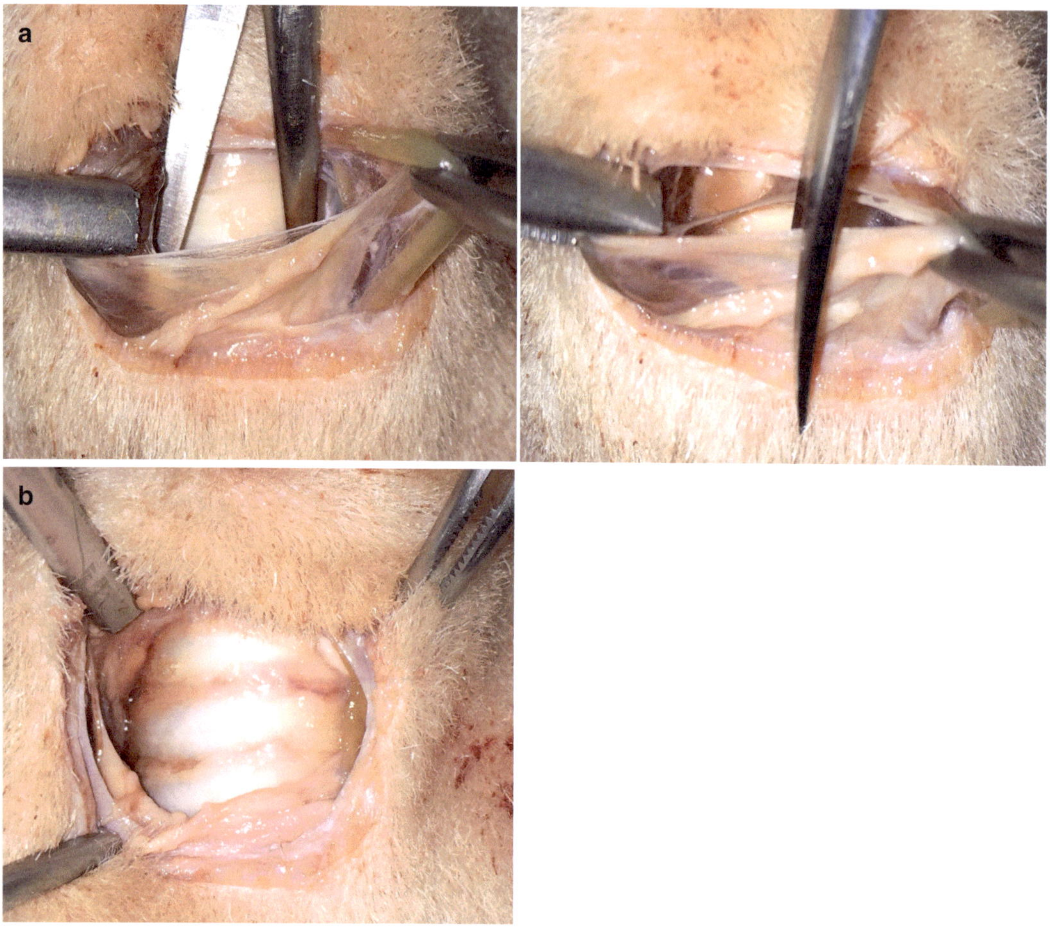

Fig. 3.5 (**a**) Strap muscle dissection. (**b**) Tracheal explosion

Step 5 Incision of the Trachea

The debate is still ongoing as to whether a vertical or horizontal tracheal incision, with or without flap, should be made. The basic principle consists of incising as few tracheal rings as possible (Figs. 3.6 and 3.7).

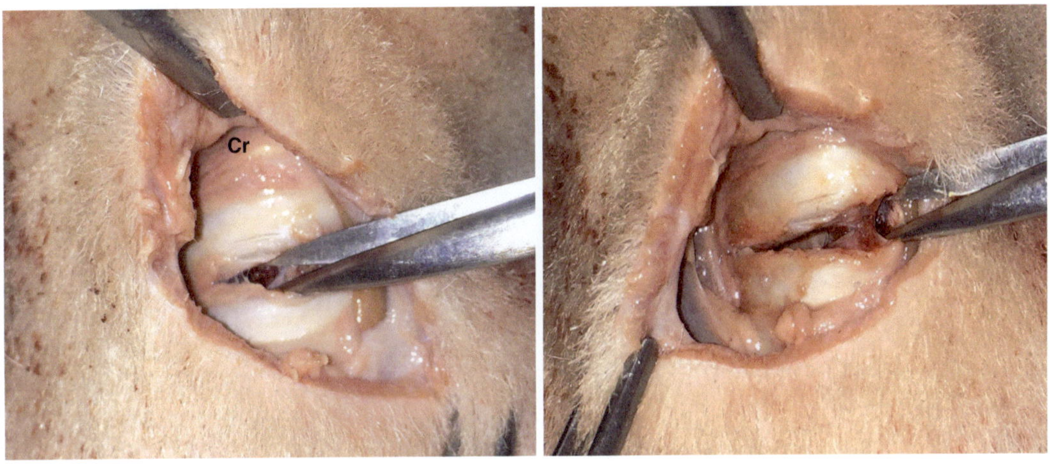

Fig. 3.6 Horizontal tracheal incision at the level of the second tracheal ring. *Cr* cricoid cartilage

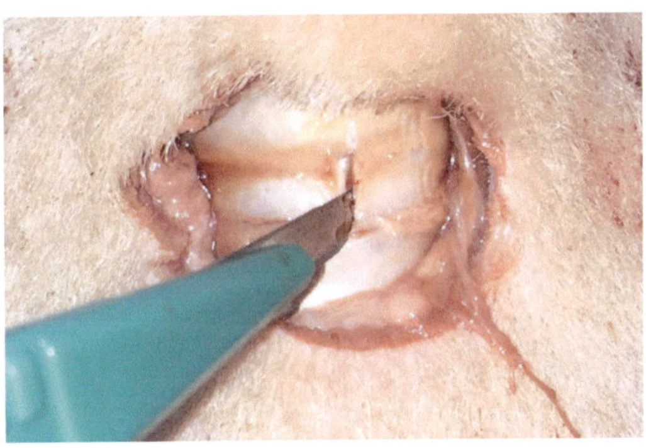

Fig. 3.7 Vertical tracheal incision

Step 6 Björk Flap Creation or Inverted H-Shaped Tracheal Opening

It is useful to use an inferiorly based Björk flap (Fig. 3.8), transecting only a single tracheal ring. You have to suture the flap to the inferior edge of the skin to facilitate reinsertion of the tracheostomy tube, while it is being changed or during accidental extubation (Fig. 3.9).

You can also create an inverted H-shaped incision, transecting only a single tracheal ring (Fig. 3.10) or two tracheal rings and reflecting tracheal flaps laterally (Fig. 3.11).

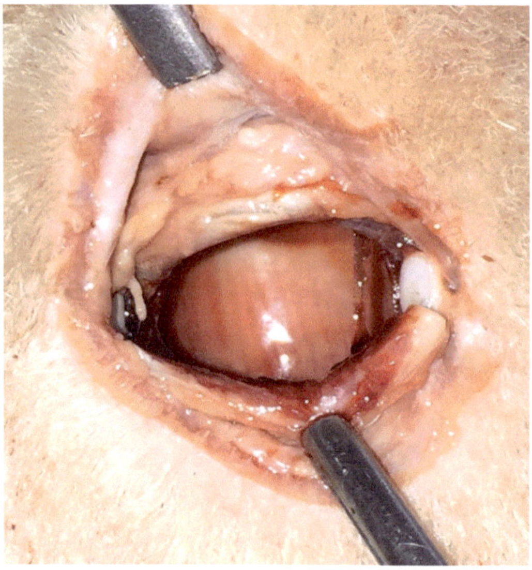

Fig. 3.8 Björk flap

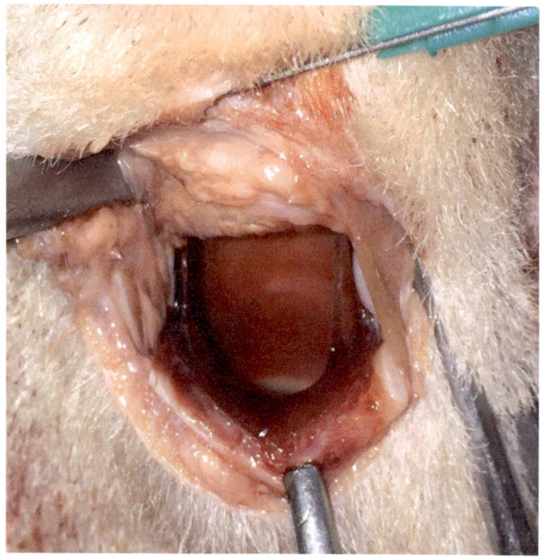

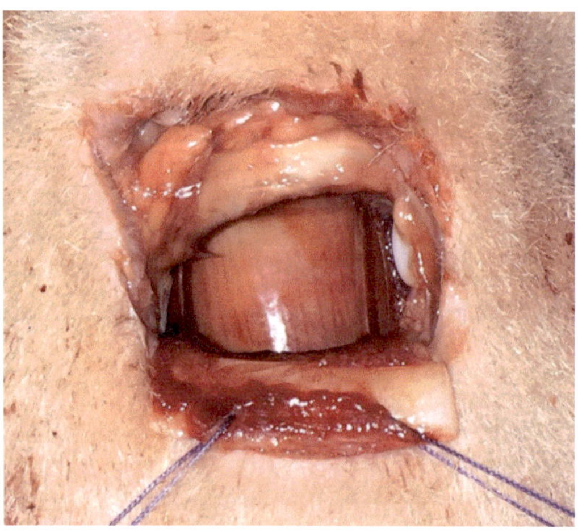

Fig. 3.9 The rest of the skin is sutured around the small tracheal opening

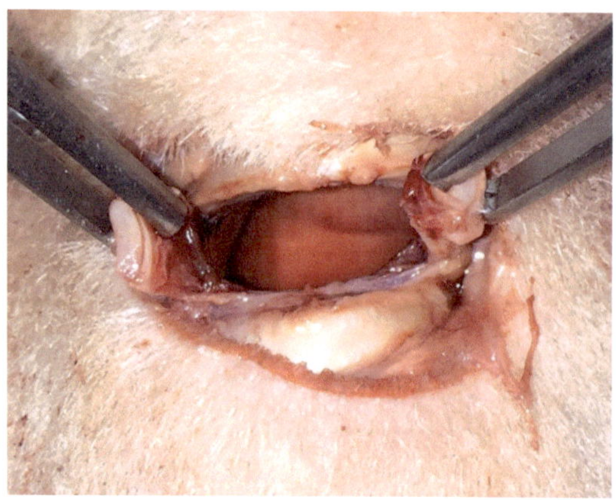

Fig. 3.10 Inverted H-shaped tracheal opening transecting only a single tracheal ring

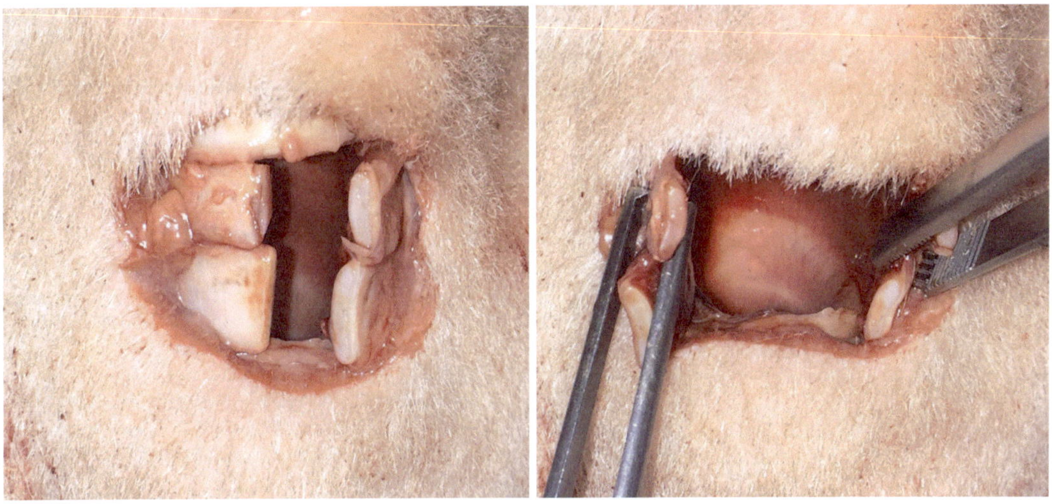

Fig. 3.11 Inverted H-shaped tracheal opening transecting two tracheal rings

Step 7 Insertion of Tracheal Cannula

An appropriately sized cannula is inserted with a tapered introducer that slightly dilates the new tracheal stoma (Fig. 3.12).

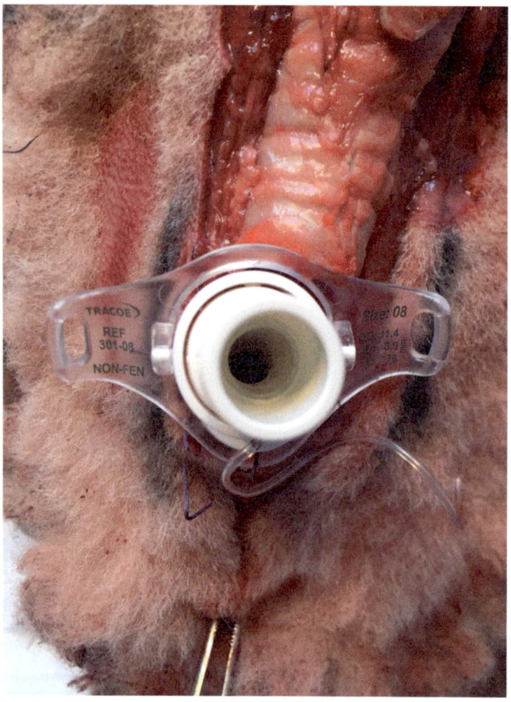

Fig. 3.12 The cannula calibrates the opening to its own size

> **Take-Home Message**
>
> - Sheep neck has great similarities with humans in size of the organs so it represents a cheap and practical model which can be used to learn airways surgery, in particular, to perform tracheotomy.

References

1. Patel SA, Meyer TK (2014) Surgical airway. Int J Crit Illn Inj Sci 4(Issue 1):71–76
2. Allen MS (2015) Surgery of the trachea. Korean J Thorac Cardiovasc Surg 48:231–237
3. Ludwing C et al (2005) Resistance to pressure of the stump after mechanical stapling or manual suture. An experimental study on sheep main bronchus. Eur J Cardiothorac Surg 27:693–696
4. Lipert D et al (2014) Care of pediatric tracheostomy in the immediate postoperative period and timing of first tube change. Int J Pediatr Otorhinolaryngol 78(12):2281–2285
5. Liu X et al (2014) The effect of early and late tracheotomy on outcomes in patients:a systematic review and cumulative metaanalysis. Otolaryngol Head Neck Surg 151(6):916–922
6. Braune S, Kluge S (2014) Airway management. Dtsch Med Wochenschr 139(40):2003–2005
7. Deprugney G, Gomez E (2014) Prevention of complications in tracheotomized patients. Rev Infirm 200: 53–54
8. Cherniack RM (1965) Tracheostomy and its management. Can Anaesth Soc J 12(4):386–397
9. Tasini Y (1965) Tracheostomy. Boll Inf Consoc Naz (Rome) 18(6):12–18
10. Monnier P (ed) (2011) Pediatric airway surgery. Springer, Heidelberg

4 Laryngotracheoplasty (Anterior and Posterior Cricoid Split)

M. Ghirelli, E. Aggazzotti Cavazza, F. Mattioli, A. Ghidini, S. Bottero, and L. Presutti

4.1 Laryngotracheal Reconstruction with Graft Expansions

Laryngotracheal reconstruction (LTR) is based on surgical principles of laryngotracheoplasty, that is:

- Enlarging the subglottic lumen by vertical incision of the anterior
- Posterior cricoid ring and splinting this

but comprises two relevant modifications:

- Subglottic airways are expanded with graft interposition.
- Cicatricial tissue is not resected in order to provide a better reepithelization during healing periods.

Fearon and Cotton since 1972 [1] with animal studies start the codification of LTR with graft expansion. In 1978 same author published the first experience of LTR with anterior costal cartilage graft (ACCG) and provided a detailed description of LTR with ACCG, reporting his experience with 11 reconstructions using the autogenous costal cartilage method [2].

Cotton described in 1984 [3] first 100 cases of LTR with anterior and posterior firmly advocating the costal cartilage graft (CCG).

This chapter described:

- *LTR with anterior graft and partial laryngofissure*
- *LTR with posterior graft full laryngofissure*

4.1.1 Instrumentation and Equipment

If possible it is better to work in pairs.

Before starting your laboratory session, you should have these materials on hand (Fig. 4.1):

- Dissection tray or a diaper
- Dissection tools: scalpel N°15 and 11 (a); needle driver (b); surgical and anatomic forceps (c); small curved mosquito forceps (d); Kocher's forceps (e); Mayo, curved, and straight iris scissors (f); suture threads 1, 0, 2–0, 3–0, 4–0 (g); Killian's speculum (h); small retractors (i); and a suction cannula(j)
- Medical gauzes (k)
- Paper towel

M. Ghirelli (✉) • E. Aggazzotti Cavazza • F. Mattioli
A. Ghidini • L. Presutti
Head and Neck Department, University Hospital of Modena, Modena, Italy
e-mail: michael.ghirelli@gmail.com

S. Bottero
Airway Surgery Unit, Laryngotracheal Team Director, Bambino Gesù Children's Hospital, Rome, Italy

A. Ghidini et al. (eds.), *Atlas of Airway Surgery*, DOI 10.1007/978-3-319-49739-6_4

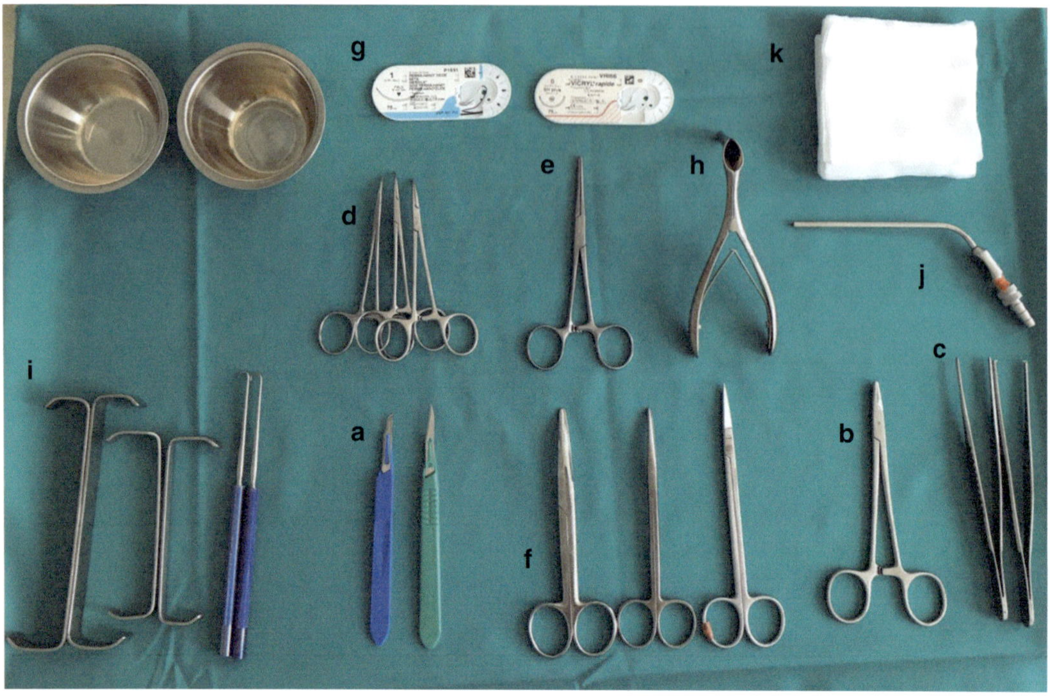

Fig. 4.1 (**a**) Scalpel N°15 and 11, (**b**) needle driver, (**c**) surgical and anatomic forceps, (**d**) small curved mosquito forceps, (**e**) Kocher's forceps, (**f**) Mayo, curved, and straight iris scissors, (**g**) suture threads 1, 0, 2–0, 3–0, 4–0, (**h**) Killian's speculum, (**i**) small retractors, and (**j**) a suction cannula

4.2 LTR with Anterior Graft Expansion

4.2.1 Indications

Isolated grade I and II subglottic stenosis (SGS).

Isolated minor grade III SGS: in these cases anterior graft (AG) is combined with a posterior costal cartilage graft PCCG.

4.3 Surgical Training Step by Step

Step 1 Skin Landmarks Identification

Recognition of the main landmarks on the skin (Fig. 4.2) is probably the most simple and fundamental step in all surgical head and neck procedures. Identification by palpation of laryngeal framework in sheep animal model is quite similar to human. In order to start the procedure, it is useful to identify superficial landmarks (Fig. 4.2):

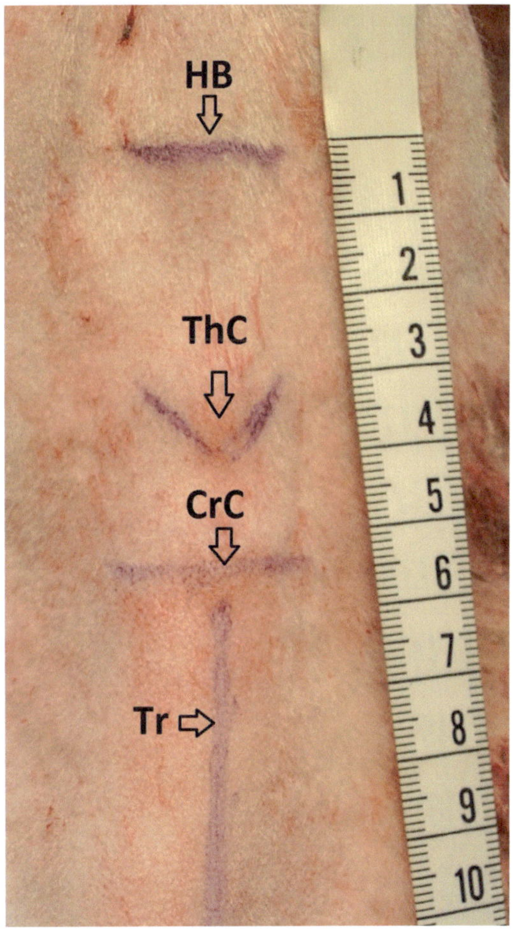

Fig. 4.2 Superficial landmarks identification. *HB* hyoid bone, partial cover by the muscles, *ThC* thyroid cartilage, *CrC* cricoid cartilage, *Tr* trachea

Step 2 Superficial Layer Dissection
Make a vertical incision about 13 cm in order to show the superficial fascia that covers muscles of the neck. Incision could be performed with 10 or 15 blades. In this step the main goal is to elevate only a cutaneous and subcutaneous flap. When all superficial fascias are exposed, surgeons have to dissect it on the midline with surgical scissors or blade. After this, to allow a good exposition of the main structures below, it is useful to suture subcutaneous tissue at the lateral skin in its upper and lower part (Fig. 4.3).

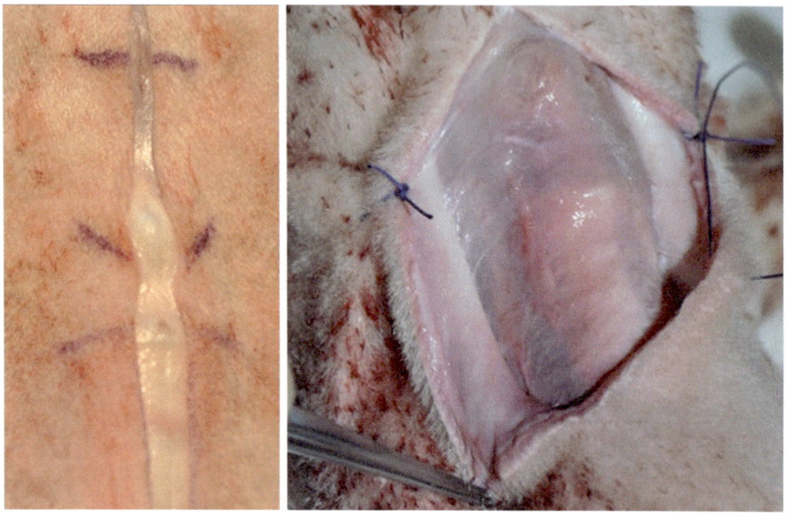

Fig. 4.3 Skin incision; superficial cervical fascia dissected and sutured with subcutaneous tissue. Below laryngeal's structures covered by its fascia

Step 3 Laryngeal Framework Identification
When the dissection of the superficial layers is completed, it is important to identify the main structures of laryngeal framework and muscles that surround it (Fig. 4.4).

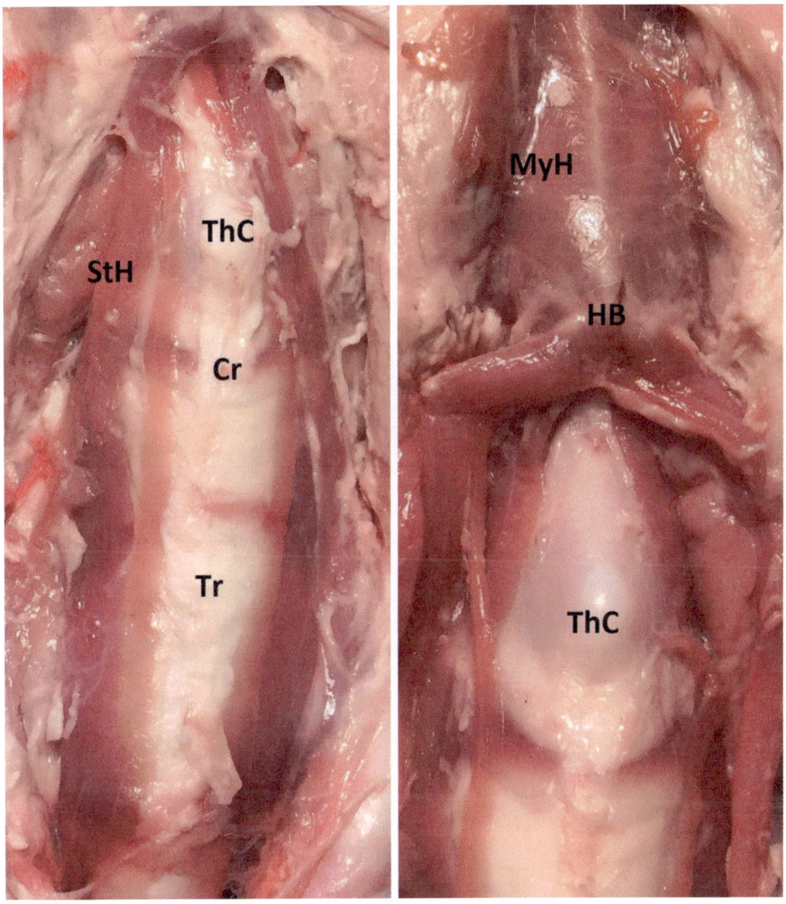

Fig. 4.4 Larynx expose with muscles surround it. *MyH* mylohyoid muscle, *HB* hyoid bone, partial cover by the muscles, *StH* sternohyoid muscle, *ThC* thyroid cartilage, *Cr* cricoid cartilage, *Tr* trachea

Step 4 Surface Marking for the Anterior Commissure

After the identification of thyroid and cricoid cartilage with ruler and dermographic pen, sign the midline. As described in comparison anatomy, the position of anterior commissure (AC) in sheep larynx is quite similar to humans; the AC is located at the midpoint of the line between the thyroid notch and inferior border of the thyroid cartilage (Fig. 4.5).

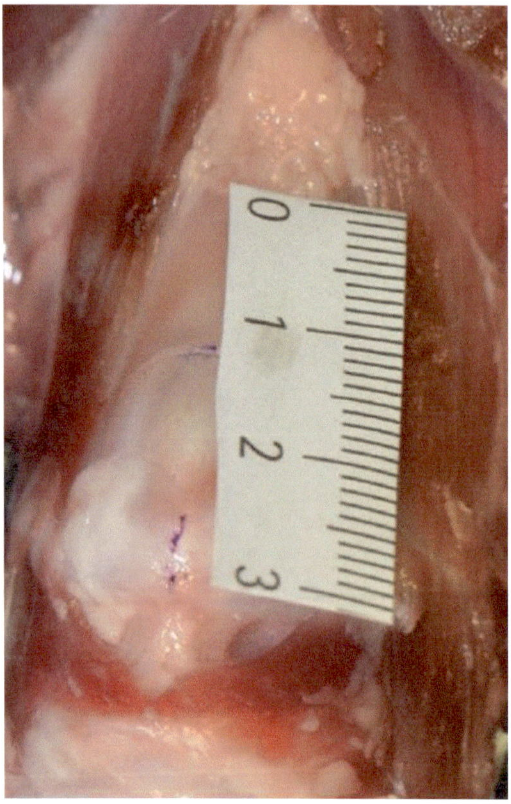

Fig. 4.5 Identification of thyroid cartilage midline and incision line identification (Gently given by Prof. Sandu)

Step 5 Partial Laryngotracheal Fissure

Normally the length of vertical incision depends on extension of stenosis evaluated in preoperative endoscopic examination. The incision performed with 15 scalpels typically extends through the lower third of the thyroid cartilage (preserving the anterior commissure), the cricothyroid membrane, the anterior cricoid arch, and the upper two tracheal rings. It is useful to preserve the cricothyroid muscles. Full laryngofissure could increase the risk of destabilizing the laryngeal framework. Measure the length and width of the desired anterior expansion graft. It is mandatory to avoid off-midline incision in order to prevent incision and damage of vocal folds (VFs) (Fig. 4.6).

At the beginning you can try the same surgical step creating a tracheo-fissure in the lower trachea, to get confidence in this technique (Fig. 4.7).

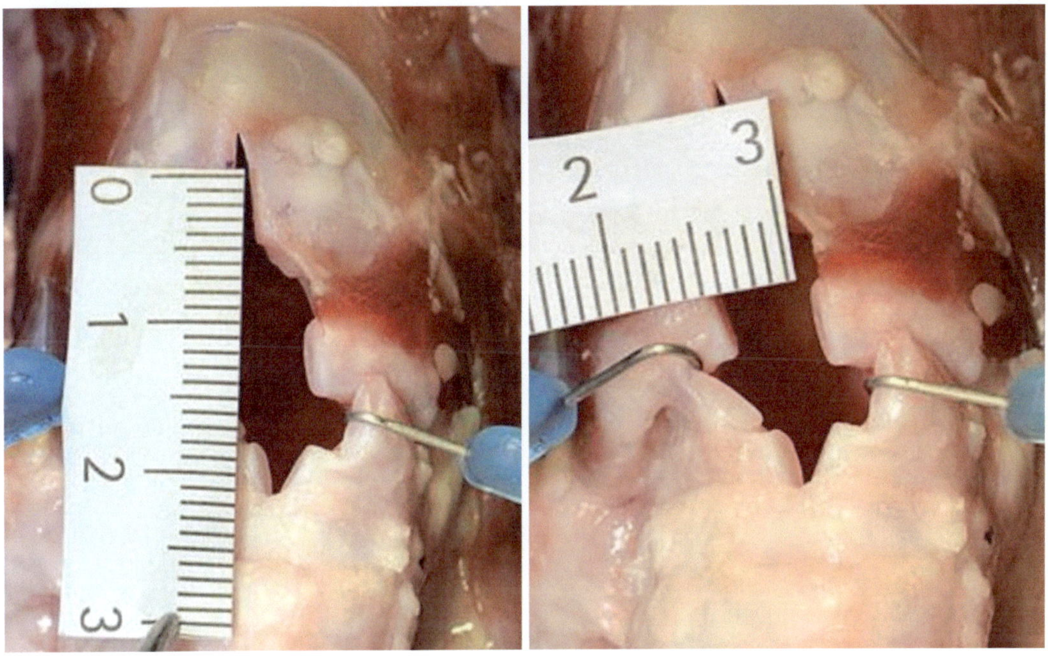

Fig. 4.6 Anterior partial laryngofissure. Measure of the length and width in order to tailor the graft (Pictures gently given by Prof. K. Sandu)

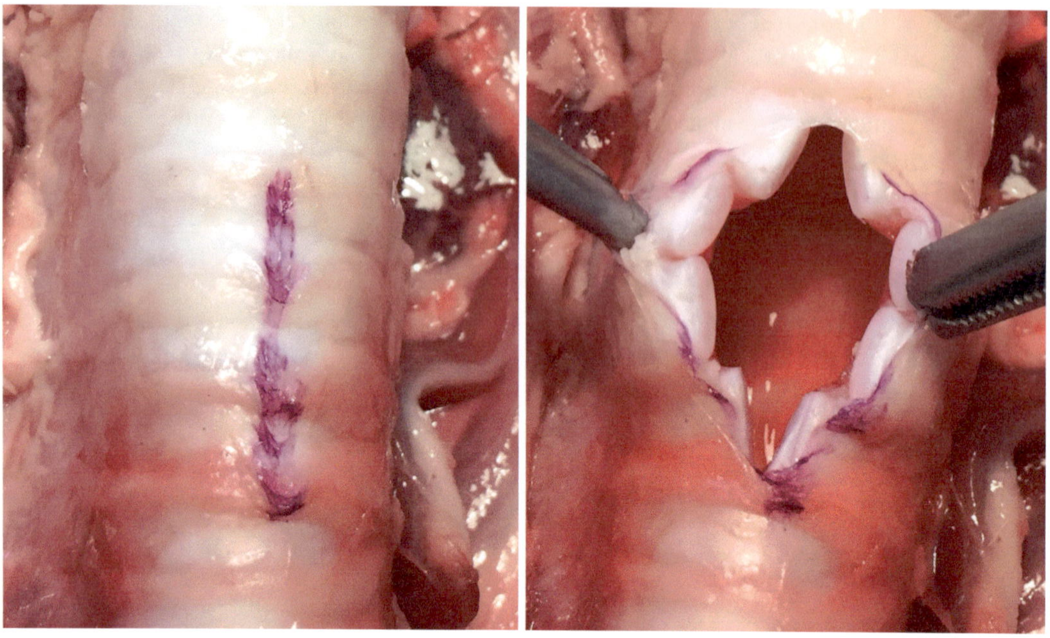

Fig. 4.7 Identification of trachea midline. Vertical incision of anterior tracheal wall

Step 6 How to Prepare Anterior Graft
In human procedure from 1970, several grafting materials were tested:

- Nasal septal cartilage
- Mucoperichondrial grafts from the nasal septum auricular cartilage
- Hyoid bone
- Thyroid cartilage
- Costal cartilage [4–6]

Costal cartilage is considered the best grafting material, due to its rigidity and availability in large quantities [2, 7].

Thyroid cartilage is preferred as graft material following an anterior cricoid split in premature neonates who have failed multiple extubation attempt [8].

For surgical training it is possible to use Fig. 4.8.

- Animal costal cartilage graft
- Eraser
- Lower tracheal wall

The Eraser, in our opinion is the better material for surgical training because is simple to shape and has low cost.

The shaping start on one side of the eraser or the perichondrial side in case of cartilage graft; a boat-shaped template is drawn to match exactly the anterior laryngeal defect, preserving superior, inferior, and lateral flanges (Fig. 4.9).

- The thickness of the carved portion of the graft must match exactly with that of the cricoid arch and trachea (Fig. 4.10).
- The thickness of the flanges can be about 2 mm (or sometimes more as flanges will remain external to the airway lumen and might undergo some degree of resorption).

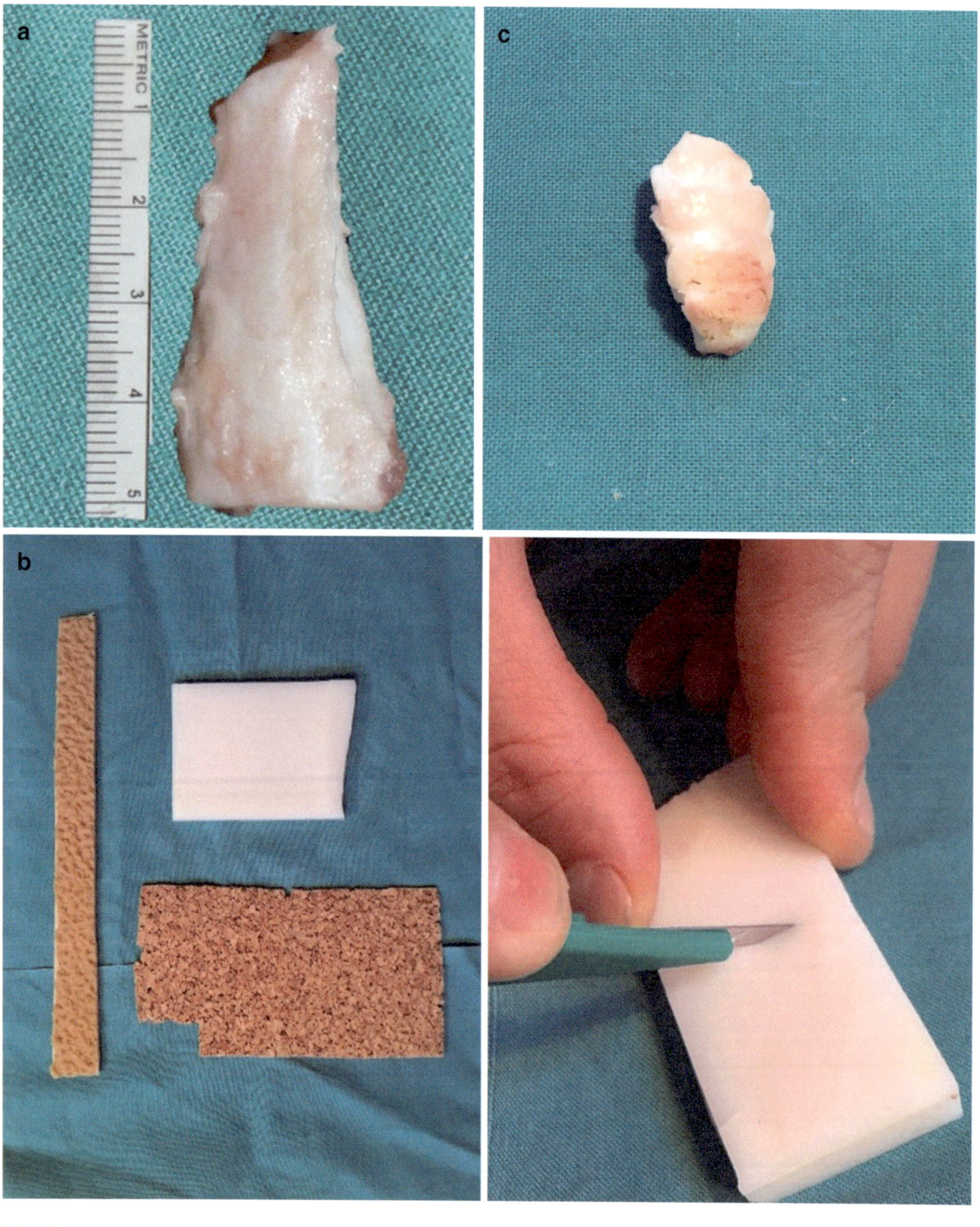

Fig. 4.8 (**a**) Costal cartilage graft, (**b**) eraser, (**c**) lower tracheal wall

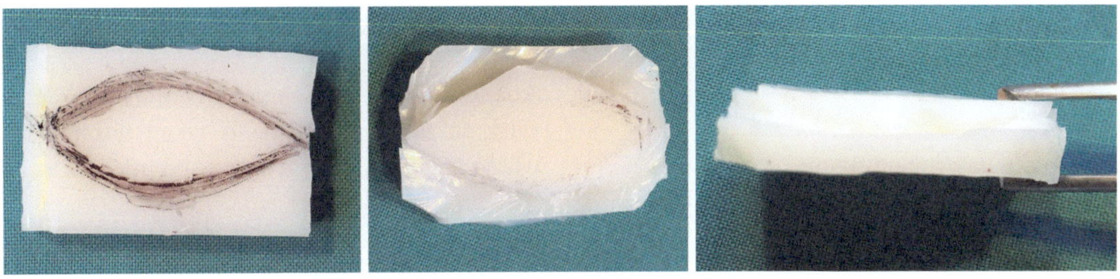

Fig. 4.9 Shaping of anterior graft, step by step

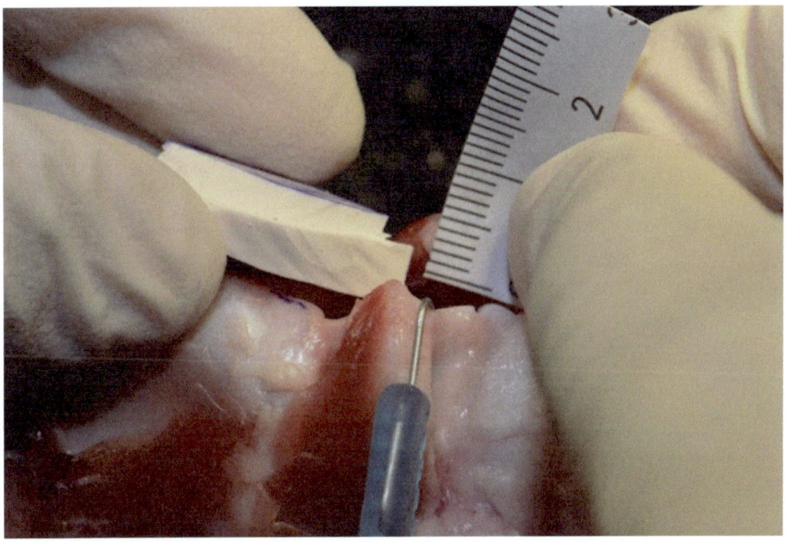

Fig. 4.10 Evaluation of graft thickness in comparison with cricoid arch and trachea (Picture gently given by Prof. K. Sandu)

Step 7 How to Suture the Anterior Graft
There are two options to suture the graft on the defect:

- Simple interrupted suture
- Horizontal mattress suture

4.3.1 Simple Interrupted Suture

The stitch (4.0 Vicryl) is inserted through the dorsal portion of the cartilage and must emerge exactly at the edge of the perichondrium on the boat-shaped portion of the graft. Depending on the length of the defect, 8–10 stitches are placed all around the graft (Figs. 4.11, 4.12, 4.13, 4.14, and 4.15).

Simple interrupted suture performed on anterior tracheal wall is a good exercise to improve suture technique (Fig. 4.16).

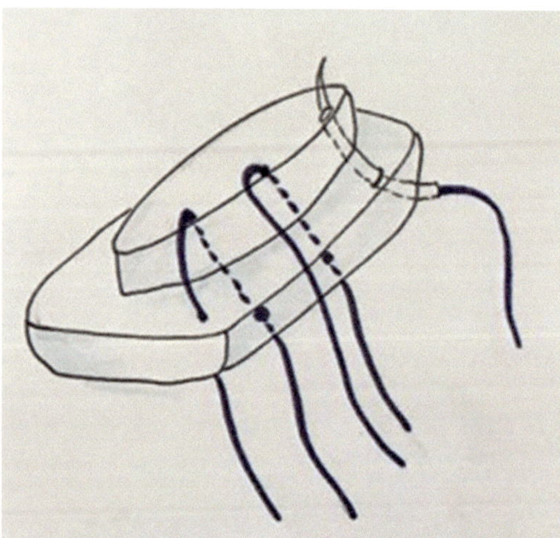

Fig. 4.11 Scheme of stitches on anterior graft

4.3.2 Horizontal Mattress Suture

An *outside-to-inside* stitch emerging submucosally on the cricoid side is taken through the whole thickness of the cricoid and tracheal wall.

- The needle is then passed from the edge of the perichondrial boat-shaped side to the dorsal part of the graft and is again reinserted 2 or 3 mm apart to emerge again at the edge of the perichondrial side (Fig. 4.17a,b).
- It is then passed again submucosally through the whole thickness of the cricoid arch or tracheal ring (Fig. 4.17c).
- The knot is tied on the outer surface of the cricoid or trachea (Fig. 4.18).

Endoscopic examination shows the correct position of graft (Fig. 4.19).

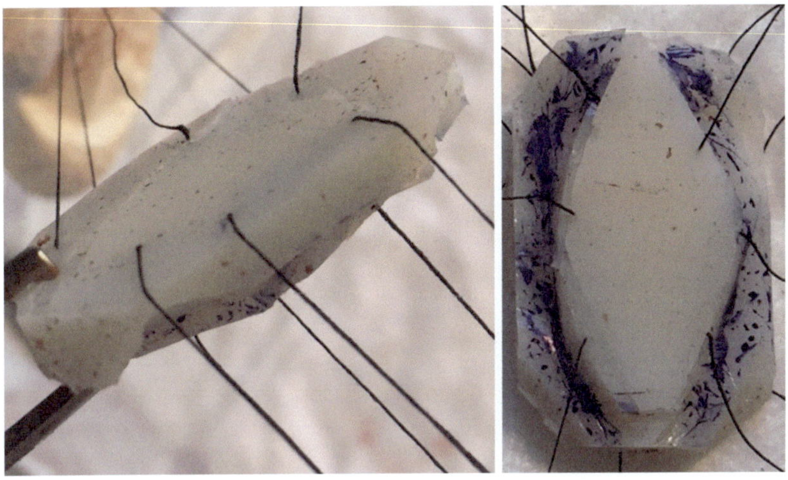

Fig. 4.12 Interrupted stitches positioning on anterior graft

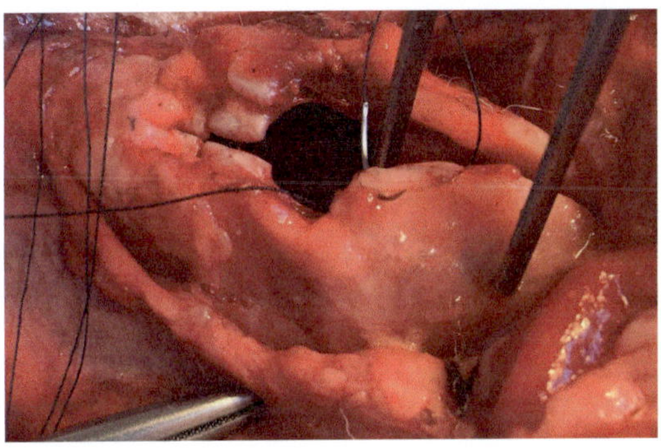

Fig. 4.13 After graft step stitches have to be positioned on anterior laryngeal split

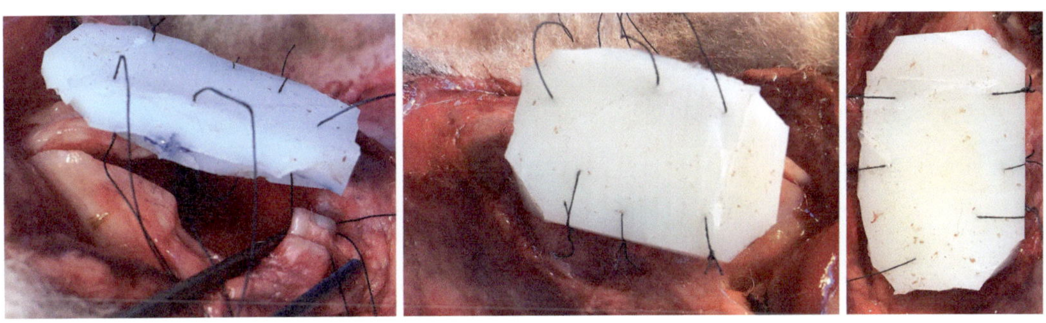

Fig. 4.14 Step-by-step stitches positioning

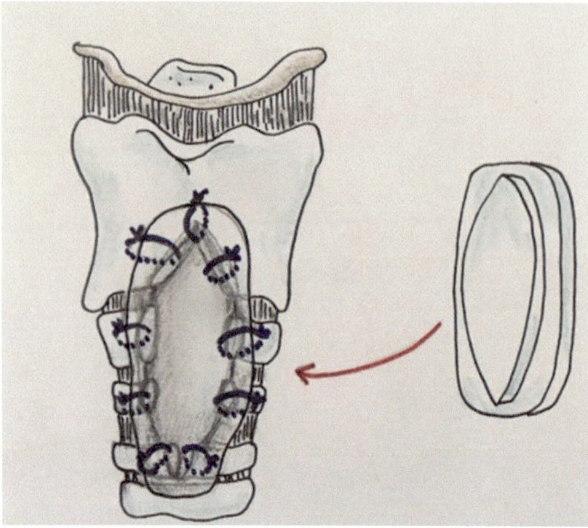

Fig. 4.15 Scheme of interrupted suture of anterior graft

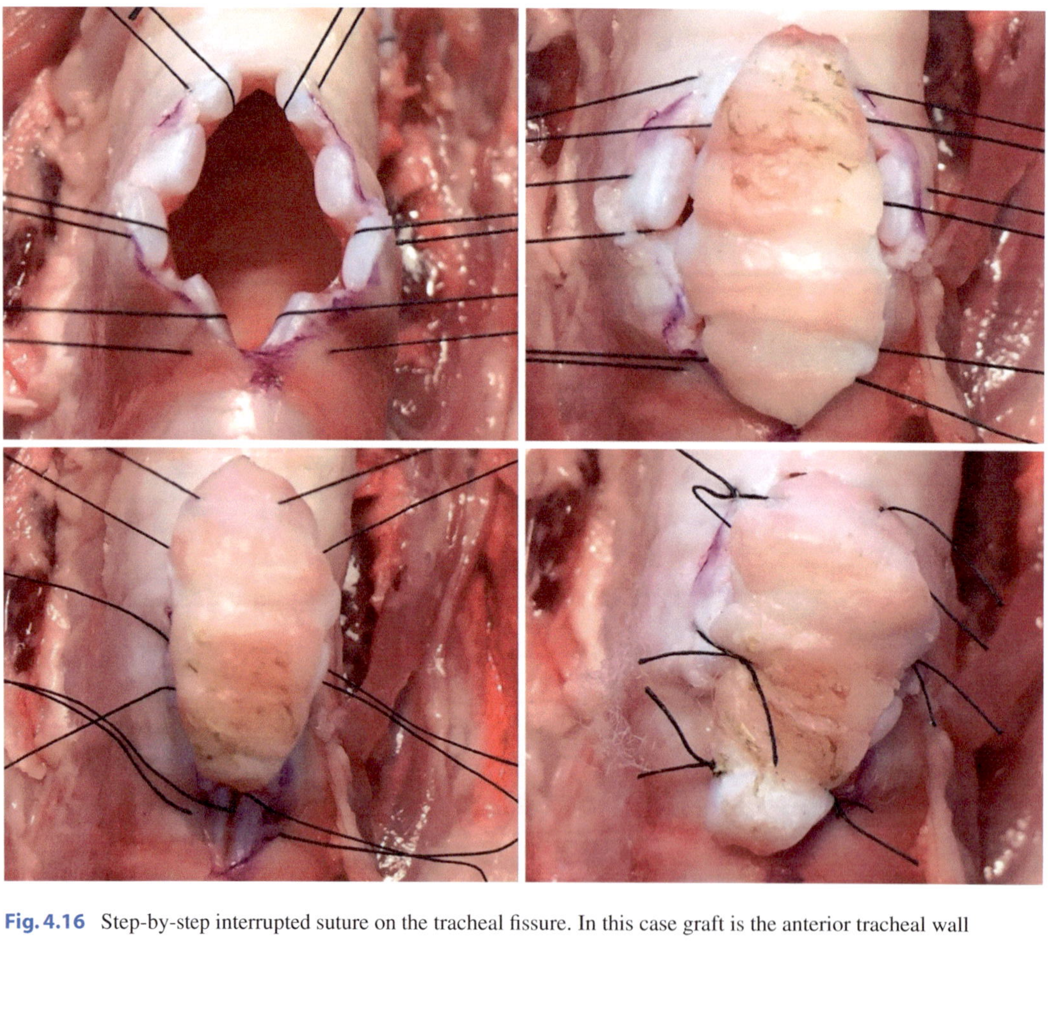

Fig. 4.16 Step-by-step interrupted suture on the tracheal fissure. In this case graft is the anterior tracheal wall

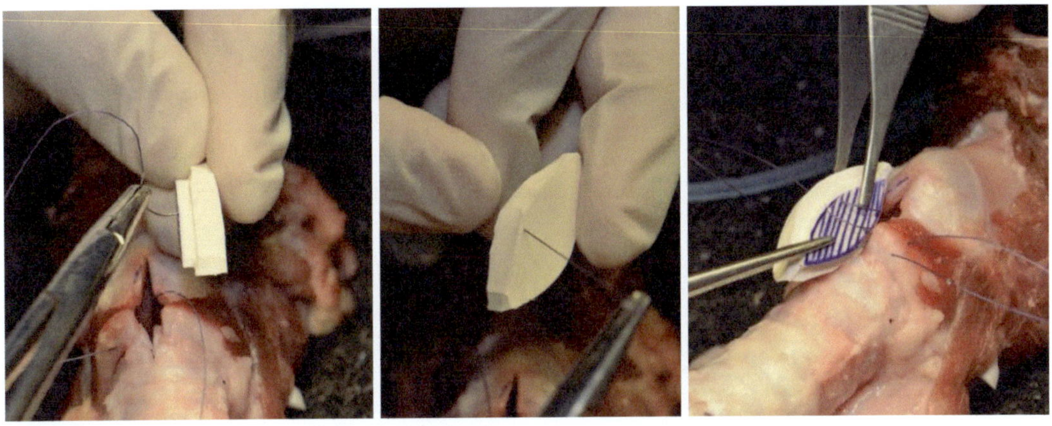

Fig. 4.17 Step-by-step horizontal mattress suture (Pictures gently given by Prof. K. Sandu)

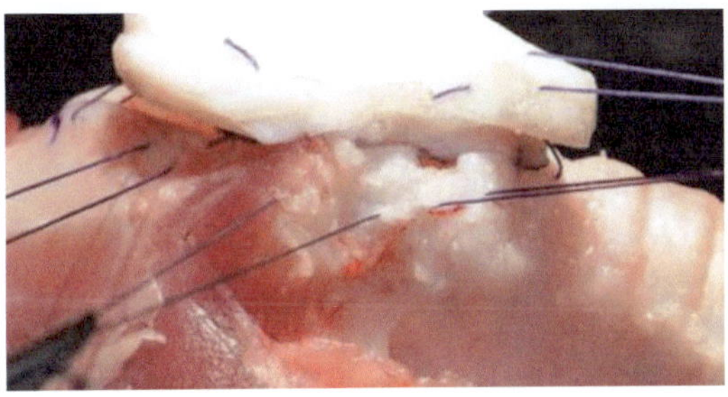

Fig. 4.18 Horizontal mattress suture allows a better contact between strap muscle and graft in order to improve revascularization (Picture gently given by Prof. K. Sandu)

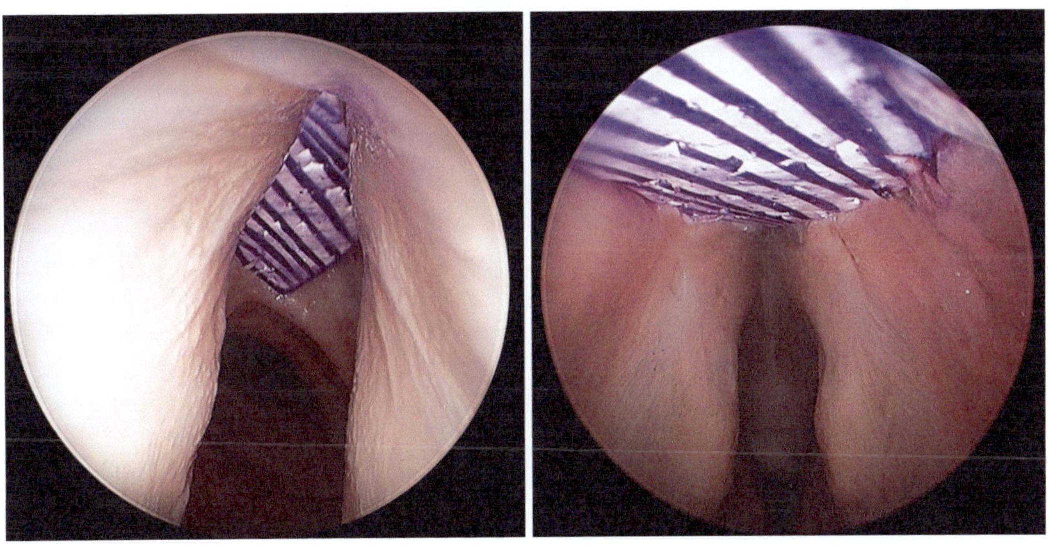

Fig. 4.19 Endoscopic view after anterior graft positioning (Pictures gently given by Prof. K. Sandu)

4.4 LTR with Posterior Graft Full Laryngofissure

4.4.1 Indication

- Every condition that requires expansion of the interarytenoid space:
- Posterior glottic stenosis (PGS) or extensive vocal fold (VF) webbing or VF synechia
- Isolated grade I, II, and possibly minor grade III subglottic stenosis in the pediatric age group

Step 5 Full Laryngotracheal Fissure
The incision extends from inferior border of thyroid cartilage up to the thyroid notch.

It is mandatory to avoid the vocal folds (VFs) and the anterior commissure.

The incision extends inferiorly including the first and second tracheal rings (Fig. 4.20).

After anterior split of cricoid and thyroid cartilage, it is necessary to suture vocal ligament with anterior commissure.

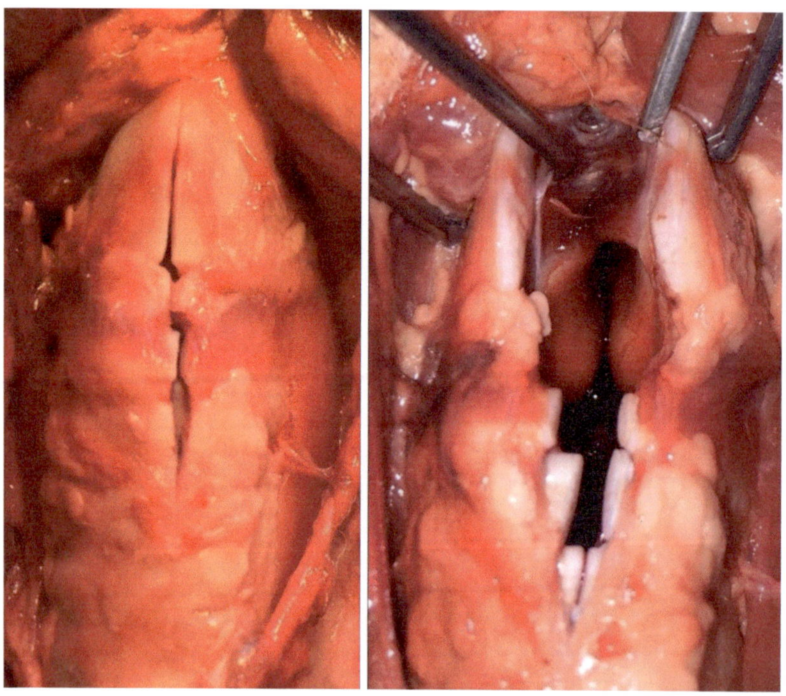

Fig. 4.20 Full laryngotracheal fissure is mandatory to maintain the midline and identify vocal folds and anterior commissure

Step 6 How to Prepare Posterior Graft
Perform a rectangular shape on one side of eraser or on perichondrium side on costal graft (Fig. 4.21).

- The length of the cranio-caudal is the same of the cricoid, and the width of the expanding cartilage normally is 5–7 mm.
- Thickness is calculated similar of the cricoid plate one.
- Lateral flanges: 2 mm extension on each side and 1–2 mm thick (Fig. 4.22).

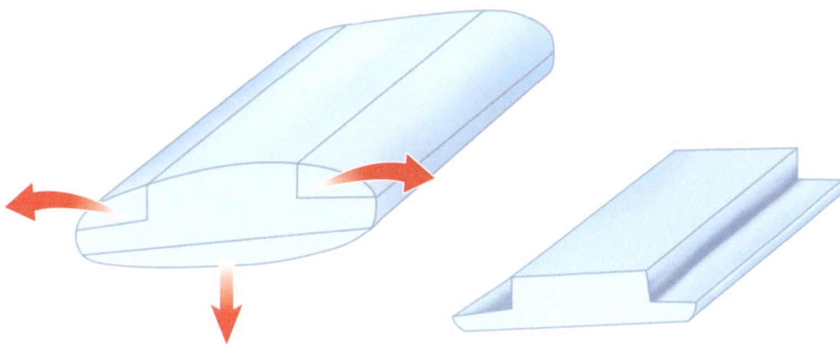

Fig. 4.21 Scheme of posterior graft shaping

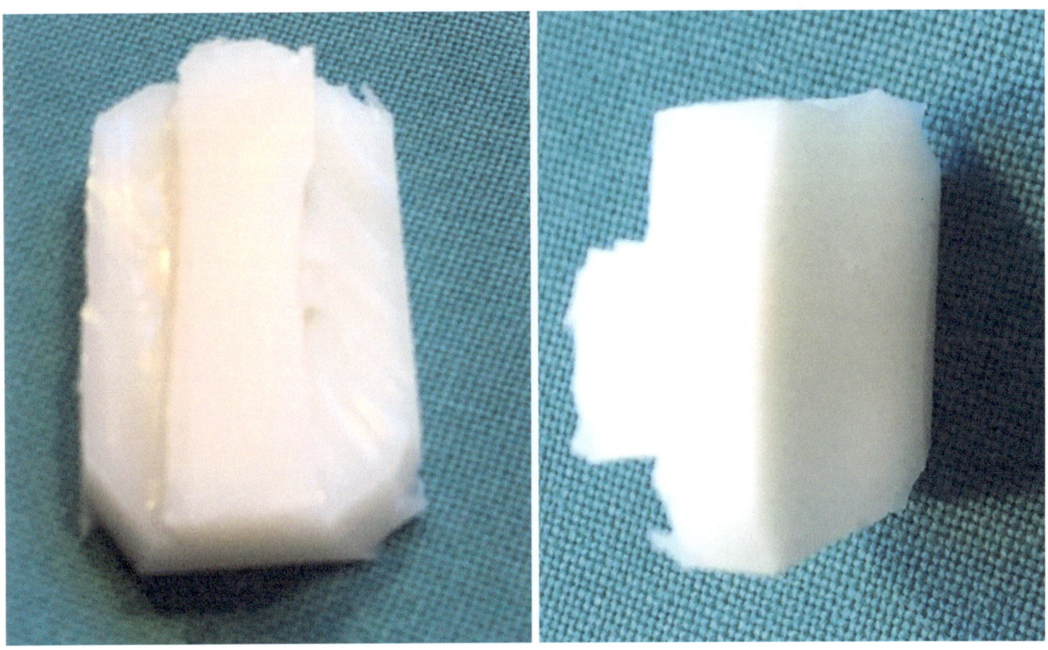

Fig. 4.22 Shaping of the posterior graft

Step 7 Posterior Cricoid Split

In this step, it is mandatory to follow up any indication because some anatomical parts are correlated with high risk of postoperative complication.

Previously, it is useful to make hydrodissection of posterior cricoid mucosa.

Divide the subglottic mucosa and posterior cricoid plate vertically in the midline with a number 15 blade to reach progressively the median raphe of the posterior cricoarytenoid muscles (Fig. 4.23a).

Be careful to avoid inadvertent incision of the retro-cricoid mucosa. Use a round knife or mosquito artery snap to split the posterior cricoid cartilage (Fig. 4.23b).

Clearly identification of the midline could be useful to avoid T off-midline incision and damage of the cricoarytenoid joints. In order to prevent this, it is useful to place a mosquito artery snap vertically behind the posterior laryngeal commissure into the pharynx and spread apart the two arytenoids.

Create two lateral pockets to insert the lateral flanges of the graft. During this step avoid posterior cricoid mucosa or esophagus injury (Fig. 4.24).

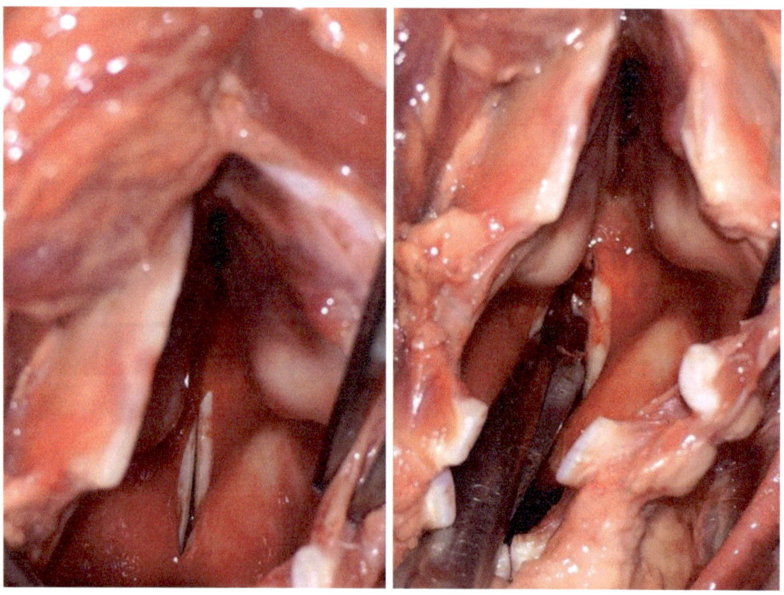

Fig. 4.23 (**a**) Mucosa and cricoid incision on the midline; (**b**) posterior cricoid splitting and evidence of posterior cricoid mucosa must be preserved

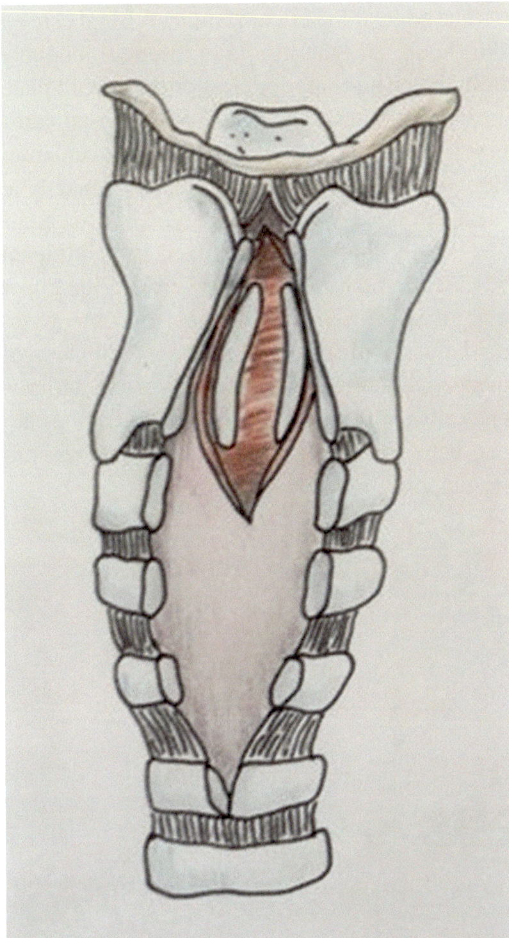

Fig. 4.24 Scheme of final result after posterior cricoid split

Step 8 Posterior Graft Positioning

The graft has to position into cricoid split and snap with lateral flanges behind cricoid cartilage splitted. Subglottic mucosa is replaced over the gap. In human procedure if the graft is too loose, it may place tissue glue (Fig. 4.25).

Graft could be sutured with cricoid cartilage. Technique consists in four stitches (4.0 Vicryl) to stabilize the graft in this way:

The needle must be inserted through the perichondrium and emerge exactly at the angle created by the lateral flanges of the cartilage (Fig. 4.26).

Correct placement of the stitches through the cricoid plate is:

The edge of the cricoid lamina is lifted using a skin hook, and the needle is inserted obliquely from the posteroinferior crest of the cricoid plate so as to fit exactly the height of the costal cartilage graft. Suture passed at the posterior and inferior crest of the cricoid plate emerging exactly at the mucosal edge (Figs. 4.27 and 4.28).

Once the graft is securely fixed, two additional 5.0 Vicryl stitches are placed between the upper margin of the graft and the posterior interarytenoid mucosa to create adequate approximation of the perichondrium with the mucosa. Similarly, one or two 5.0 stitches are also placed at the caudal edge of the graft for the same reasons (Fig. 4.29).

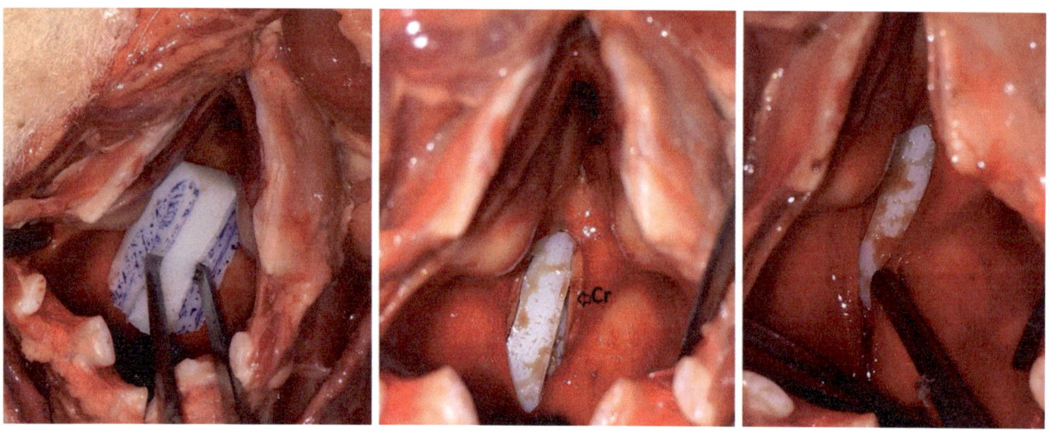

Fig. 4.25 (**a**) Posterior graft positioning; (**b**) evidence of posterior cricoid cartilage (*Cr*) and flanges correctly positioned into lateral pockets, (**c**) subglottic mucosa repositioning

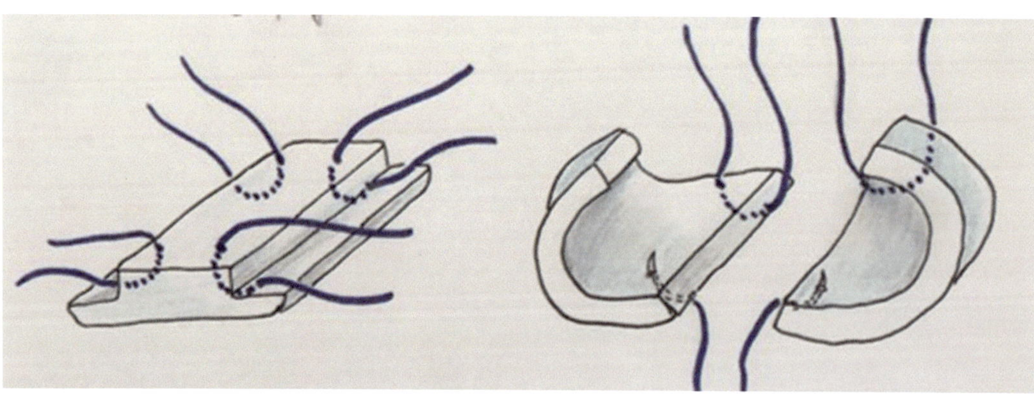

Fig. 4.26 Scheme of posterior stitches positioning technique

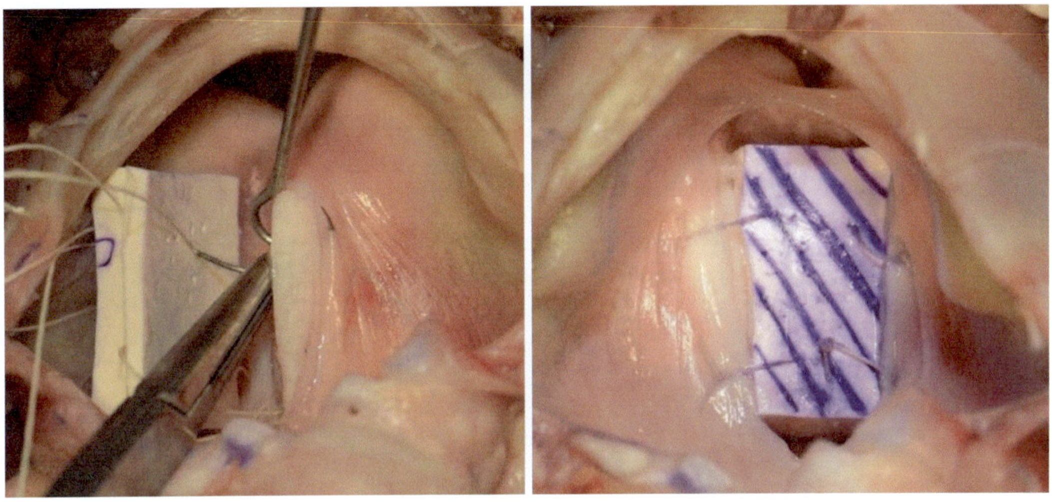

Fig. 4.27 Posterior stitches positioning technique. Note the exactly emerging at the mucosal edge (Pictures gently given by Prof. K. Sandu)

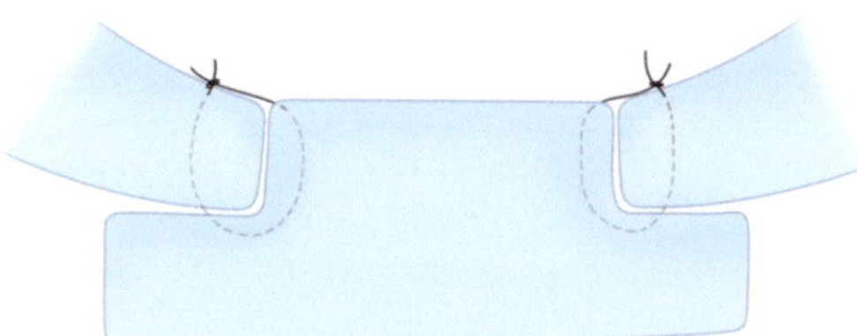

Fig. 4.28 Scheme of posterior graft interrupted suture

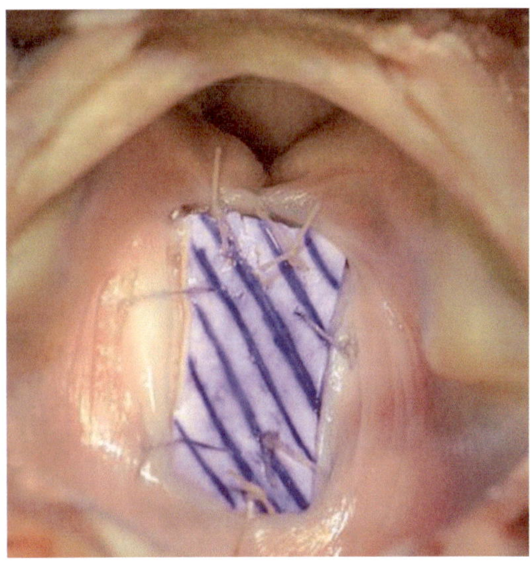

Fig. 4.29 Upper and lower stitches to conclude graft suture

Step 7 Closure of Larynx

Closure of the laryngofissure is achieved by placing first a stitch at the anterior laryngeal commissure to reposition both VFs exactly at the same level. The stitch should pass through the mucosa of the VFs to restore a sharp mucosalized anterior commissure. This is essential to preserve a good voice.

References

1. Fearon B, Cotton R (1972) Subglottic stenosis in infants and children: the clinical problem and experimental surgical correction. Can J Otolaryngol 1:281–289
2. Cotton R (1978) Management of subglottic stenosis in infancy and childhood. Review of a consecutive series of cases managed by surgical reconstruction. Ann Otol Rhinol Laryngol 87:649–657
3. Cotton RT (1984) Pediatric laryngotracheal stenosis. J Pediatr Surg 19:699–704
4. Krizek TJ, Kirchner JA (1972) Tracheal reconstruction with an autogenous mucochondrial graft. Plast Reconstr Surg 50:123–130
5. Lusk RP, Kang DR, Muntz HR (1993) Auricular cartilage grafts in laryngotracheal reconstruction. Ann Otol Rhinol Laryngol 102:247–254
6. Toohill RJ, Martinelli DL, Janowak MC (1976) Repair of laryngeal stenosis with nasal septal grafts. Ann Otol Rhinol Laryngol 85:600–608
7. Doig CM, Eckstein HB, Waterston DJ (1973) The surgical treatment of laryngeal and subglottic obstruction in infancy and childhood. Z Kinderchir Grenzgeb 12:293–303
8. Fearon B, Cinnamond M (1976) Surgical correction of subglottic stenosis of the larynx. Clinical results of the Fearon- Cotton operation. J Otolaryngol 5:475–478

5 Slide Tracheoplasty

M. Bettini, S. Bottero, F. Mattioli, A. Ghidini, and L. Presutti

> **Core Messages**
> Slide tracheoplasty is the procedure of choice for long-segment tracheal stenosis. This procedure shortens the trachea by half but doubles its circumference and quadruples its cross-sectional area.

5.1 Introduction

Slide tracheoplasty (ST), first described in 1989, has become the procedure of choice for long-segment tracheal stenosis (LSTS) with stenosis of more than 2/3 of the trachea [1].

LSTS is a severe and often life-threatening anatomical anomaly constricting the trachea for >50% of its length [2]. It is usually associated with complete tracheal rings and congenital heart defects (pulmonary artery sling is one of the more common). ST is moreover indicated for the treatment of acquired LSTS when simple resection anastomosis is deemed impossible without undue risk of anastomotic dehiscence.

The only contraindication for this procedure is the presence of a bronchus suis ("pig bronchus") with significant tracheal length between itself and the carina because it can cause a problem with mobilization of the trachea.

Although there exist several different techniques (costal cartilage tracheoplasty, pericardial patch tracheoplasty, tracheal resection, tracheal autograft tracheoplasty, and slide tracheoplasty) for management of LSTS and congenital tracheal rings, in the last decade, it has become clear that slide tracheoplasty should be the preferred option, especially in the young [3]. In fact this procedure shortens the trachea by half but doubles its circumference and quadruples its cross-sectional area [4]. Moreover one of the most important advantages of slide tracheoplasty is that the reconstruction is done with native vascularized cartilaginous trachea, which eliminates malacia and granuloma formation as postoperative complications [5].

M. Bettini (✉) • F. Mattioli • A. Ghidini • L. Presutti
Head and Neck Department, University Hospital of Modena, Modena, Italy
e-mail: margherita.bettini86@gmail.com

S. Bottero
Airway Surgery Unit, Laryngotracheal Team Director, Bambino Gesù Children's Hospital, Rome, Italy

A. Ghidini et al. (eds.), *Atlas of Airway Surgery*, DOI 10.1007/978-3-319-49739-6_5

5.2 Instrumentation and Equipment

If possible it is better to work in pairs.

Before starting your laboratory session, you should have these materials on hand (Fig. 5.1):

- Dissection tray or a diaper
- Dissection tools: scalpel N°15 and 11; needle driver; surgical and anatomic forceps; small curved mosquito forceps; Kocher's forceps; Mayo, curved, and straight iris scissors; suture threads 1,0, 2–0, 3–0, 4–0; Killian's speculum; small retractors; and a suction cannula
- Medical gauzes
- Paper towel

Set up the diaper on the bench and then the dissection tray on the diaper. Obtain dissection instruments and finally put the head into the dissection tray or on the diaper with the neck extended in the dorsal recumbent position (Fig. 5.2). The anterior part of the sheep's neck has to be previously shaved.

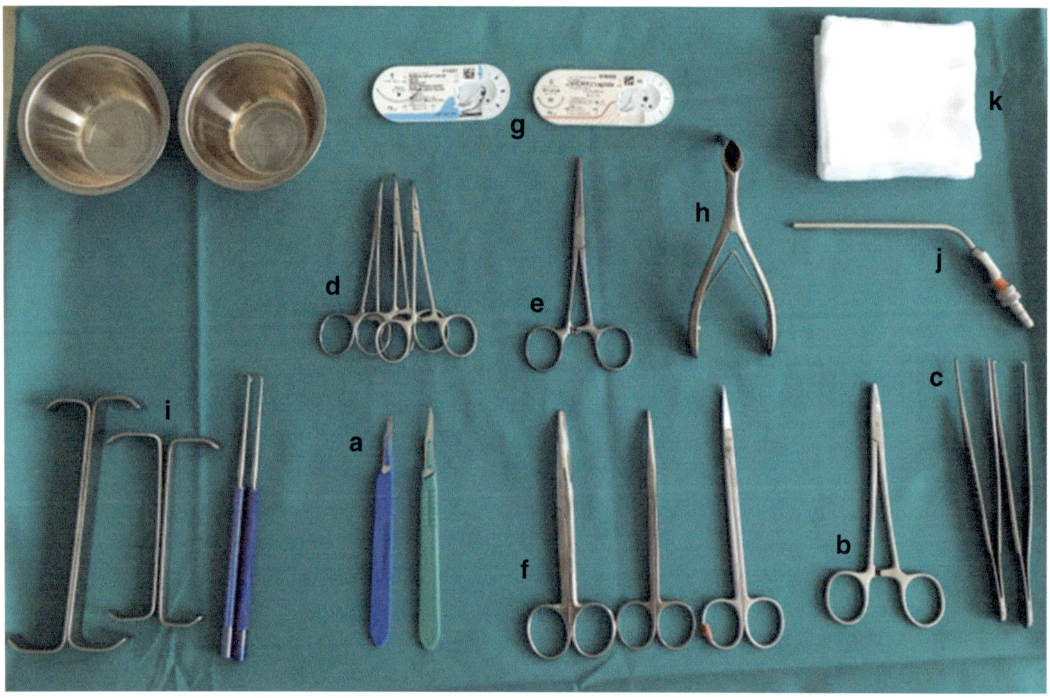

Fig. 5.1 Set of surgical instruments. *a* scalpel, *b* needle driver, *c* surgical and anatomical forceps, *d* small curved mosquito forceps, *e* Kocher's forceps, *f* scissors, *g* suture threads, *h* Killian's speculum, *i* small retractors, *j* suction cannula, *k* medical gauzes

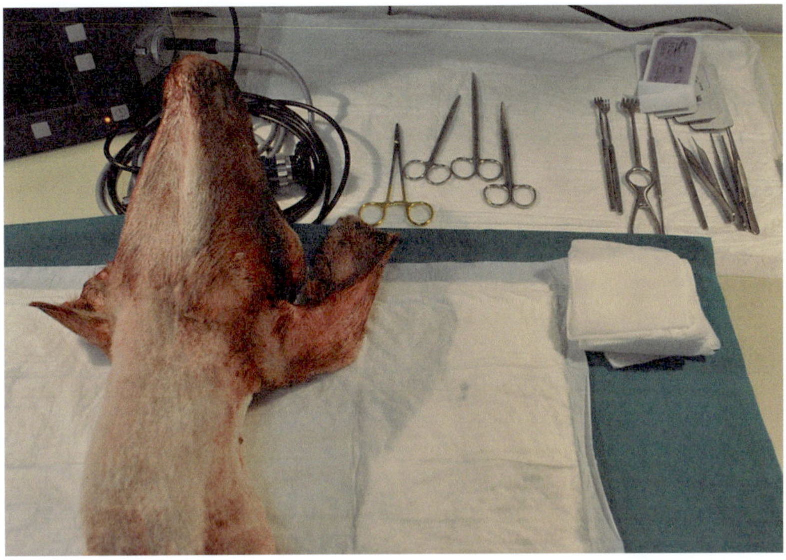

Fig. 5.2 Set-up of the surgical field

5.3 Slide Tracheoplasty

5.3.1 Skin Landmark Identification

Recognizing the main landmarks on the skin is probably the most simple and fundamental step in all surgical head and neck procedures. Identification by palpation of laryngeal framework in sheep animal model is quite similar to human.

In order to start the procedure, it is useful to identify (Fig. 5.3):

- Hyoid bone, partial cover by the muscles
- Thyroid cartilage
- Cricoid cartilage
- Trachea

5.3.2 Superficial Layer Dissection

Make a vertical incision about 13 cm in order to show the superficial fascia that covers the muscles of the neck (Fig. 5.4). Incision could be performed with 10 or 15 blade.

In this step the main goal is to elevate only a cutaneous and subcutaneous flap.

When all superficial fascia is exposed, the surgeon has to dissect it on the midline with surgical scissor or blade. After this, to allow a good exposition of the main structures below, it is useful to suture subcutaneous tissue at the lateral skin in its upper and downer part (Fig. 5.5).

5.3.3 Laryngeal Framework Identification

When the dissection of the superficial layers is completed, it is important to identify the main structures of laryngeal framework and muscles that surround it (Fig. 5.6).

5.3.4 Infrahyoid Muscle Dissection

Infrahyoid muscles are retracted laterally, resulting in optimal exposure of the lower edge of the thyroid cartilage over its entire width.

It is useful to suture the bigger muscles to subcutaneous layer in order to maintain a wide surgical field. This step simulates the strap muscle dissection on the midline performed in the human procedure in order to expose the hyoid bone and trachea. Sheep thyroid does not have an isthmus so it is not necessary to split thyroid gland on the midline (Fig. 5.7).

Now it is possible to identify all the landmarks (Fig. 5.8).

5.3.5 Dissection of the Trachea

The dissection of the trachea (Fig. 5.9) is done only anteriorly and slightly laterally without identifying the recurrent laryngeal nerves (RNLs). Surgical pearls to avoid RNL injury are:

- Stay close contact with the outer perichondrium of the tracheal rings.
- RLN identification on sheep animal model is not the goal of the procedure. In human procedure to minimize RLN injury, dissection must be carried out against the trachea without recurrent laryngeal nerve visualization.
- Avoid dissection above the posterolateral border of the cricoid plate in order to avoid injury to the RLNs.

The vascular supply of the trachea is into the tracheoesophageal groove, and it must be preserved.

In patient with LSTS, the dissection is carried on laterally over the whole distance of the stenotic segment, staying in close contact with the tracheal rings to preserve the posterolateral vascular supply to the trachea and avoid damage to recurrent laryngeal nerves.

Remarks In infants and small children, it has been possible to expose the trachea sufficiently through a collar incision alone. If additional exposure is required, the upper sternum or even the entire sternum may be divided.

5.3.6 Slide Tracheoplasty: Tracheal Transection

The most important steps of slide tracheoplasty are showed in Fig. 5.10.

The stenotic segment's length needs to be precisely measured and its midpoint marked with an intramural stitch; then the trachea is divided transversally in the mid portion of the stenosis (Fig. 5.11).

The proximal stump is freed circumferentially until the posterior membranous trachea of the first one or two normal tracheal rings is identified (Fig. 5.12). Superior mobilization in humans is routinely via the division of the thyroid isthmus (absent in sheep) or very rarely by a hyoid release. Also the caudal segment is mobilized in the same way.

Now the posterior wall of the cranial segment is incised superiorly for the length of the stenosis, while the anterior wall of the caudal segment is incised inferiorly for the length of the stenosis or until the carina, whichever is encountered first (Fig. 5.13). The reason for orienting these incisions in the proximal and distal segments is due to the fact that it would be far more difficult to access the posterior incision were it made in the distal segment.

However, K. Sandu suggests to perform the incisions in an opposite way: the cranial segment of the trachea is incised anteriorly, while the caudal segment is incised posteriorly (Fig. 5.14).

Finally the right-angled corners at the midpoint tracheal division are trimmed above and below to facilitate closure (Figs. 5.15 and 5.16).

5.3.7 Tracheal Anastomosis

The tracheal segments are then overlapped with the cranial segment placed anteriorly (Fig. 5.17).

K. Sandu performed the anastomosis, placing the cranial segment posteriorly (Fig. 5.18).

An oblique, oval-shaped anastomosis is performed with 4.0, 5.0, or 6.0 interrupted [6] or running suture technique [3].

The first stitch is placed posteriorly from the apex of the cartilaginous stump to the membranous trachea (Fig. 5.19).

Enough of the distal cartilaginous stump must be sutured posteriorly and laterally to expand the tracheal lumen as much as possible (Fig. 5.20).

The final suture being placed anteriorly (Fig. 5.21). All sutures are thrown before being tied.

Sutures are placed approximately 3 mm apart through the full thickness of the trachea so that the knots will be extraluminal (Figs. 5.22 and 5.23).

To avoid a figure-eight deformity of the reconstructed airway, the anterior tracheal segment is thus slightly intussuscepted onto the posterior tracheal segment (Fig. 5.24) on the longitudinal aspect of the anastomosis, and the distal anterior end is sutured flush to the anterior wall of the carina.

To conclude fibrin glue is placed over the anastomosis.

Remarks A leak test in humans is performed by flooding the surgical field with saline solution and performing a Valsalva to 20 cm of water pressure.

If a tracheostomy is present, and the stoma is adjacent to the stenosis, we advocate it be incorporated into the repair; otherwise it is left for conventional de-cannulation once the patient needs only minimal ventilation [2].

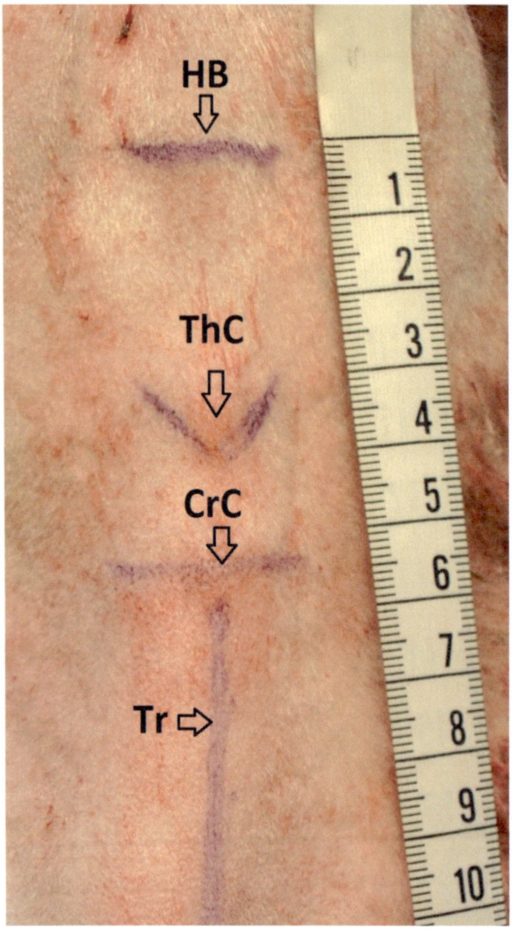

Fig. 5.3 Superficial landmark identification. *HB* hyoid bone, *ThC* thyroid cartilage, *Cr* cricoid cartilage, *Tr* trachea

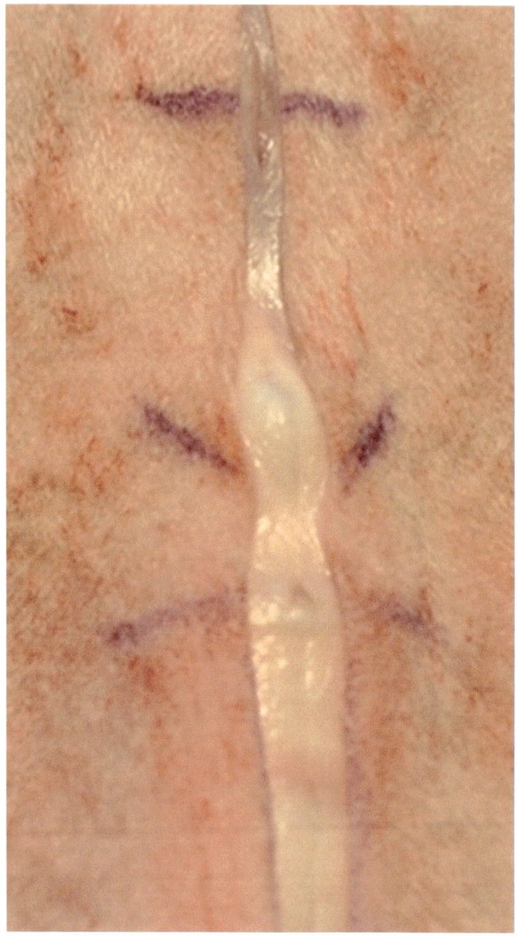

Fig. 5.4 Skin incision

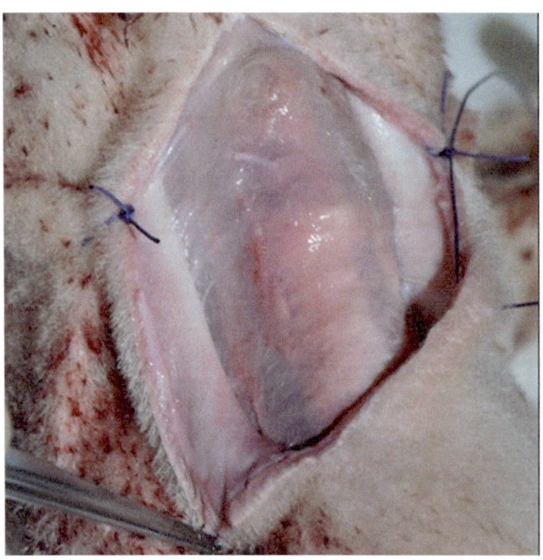

Fig. 5.5 Superficial cervical fascia dissected and sutured with subcutaneous tissue. Below, laryngeal's structures covered by its fascia

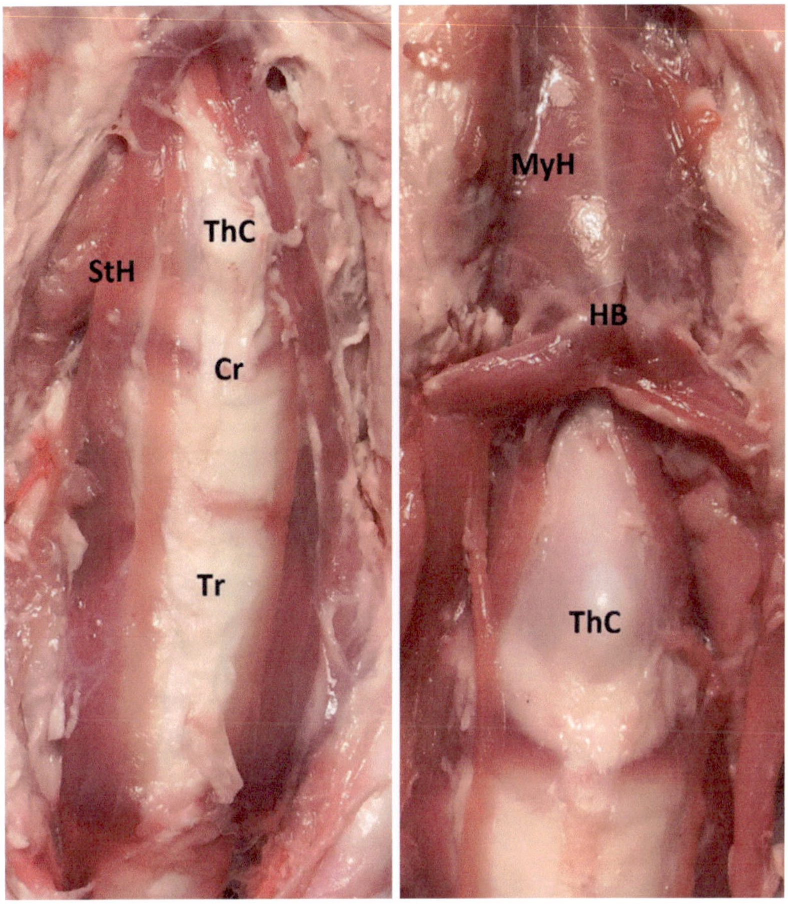

Fig. 5.6 Laryngeal framework identification. *MyH* mylohyoid muscle; *HB* hyoid bone, partial cover by the muscles; StH sternohyoid muscle; *ThC* thyroid cartilage; *Cr* cricoid cartilage; *Tr* trachea

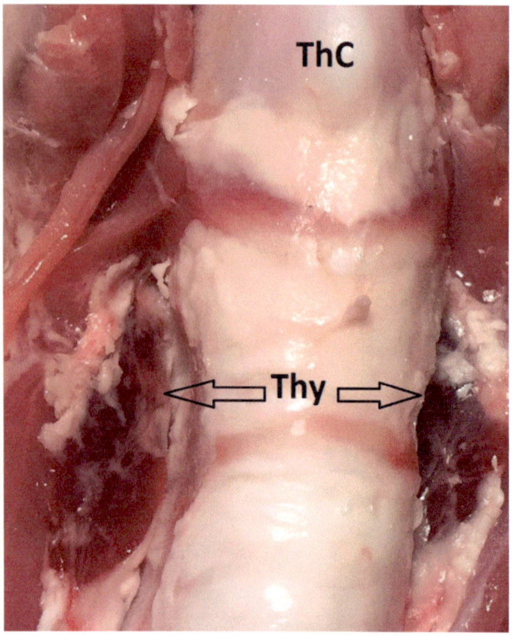

Fig. 5.7 Thyroid gland dissected. *ThC* thyroid cartilage, *Thy* thyroid gland

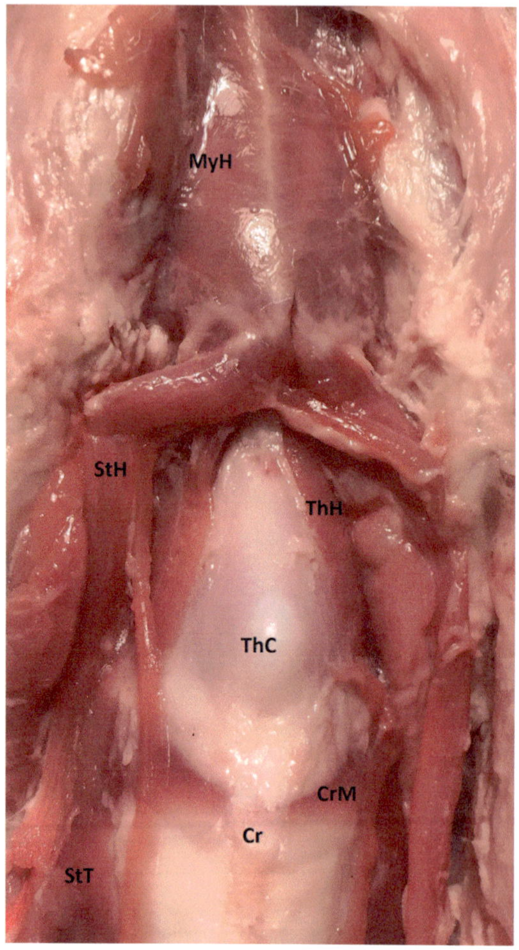

Fig. 5.8 Strap muscles dissected and mylohyoid muscle. *MyH* mylohyoid muscle, *StH* sternohyoid muscle, *ThH* thyrohyoid muscle, *StT* sternothyroid muscle, *ThC* thyroid cartilage, *Cr* cricoid cartilage, *CrM* cricothyroid muscle

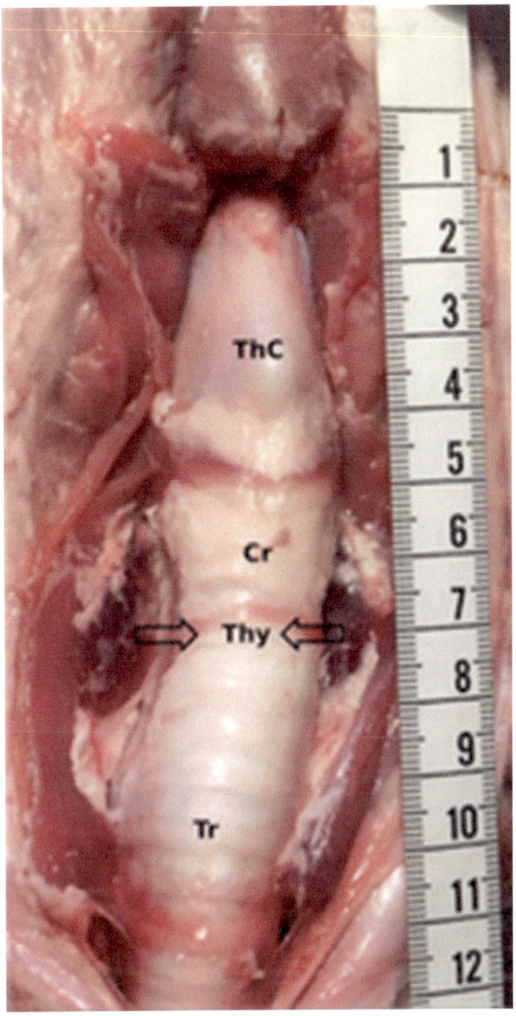

Fig. 5.9 Exposure of tracheal laryngeal axis. *ThC* thyroid cartilage, *Cr* cricoid cartilage, *Tr* trachea, *Thy* thyroid gland

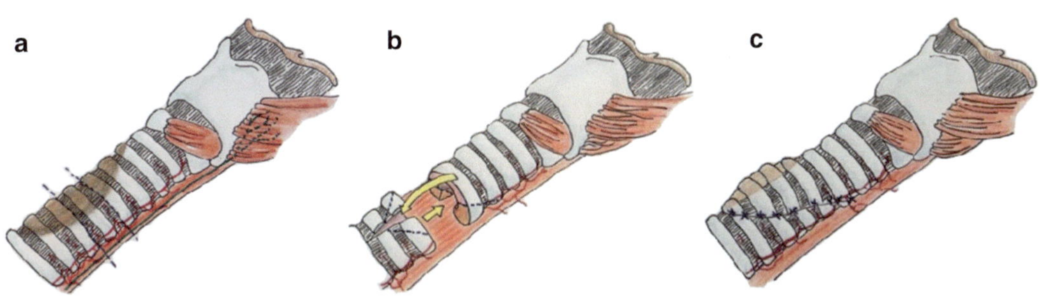

Fig. 5.10 Slide tracheoplasty. (**a**) The stenotic segment (in *brown*) is transected exactly at its midpoint. (**b**) The stenotic segment is longitudinally slit anteriorly on its caudal segment and posteriorly on its cranial segment. By gentle traction, the upper and lower segments are slid over one another. (**c**) An oval-shaped, oblique anastomosis from posterior to anterior is made, thereby shortening the trachea by half and increasing its cross-sectional area by four

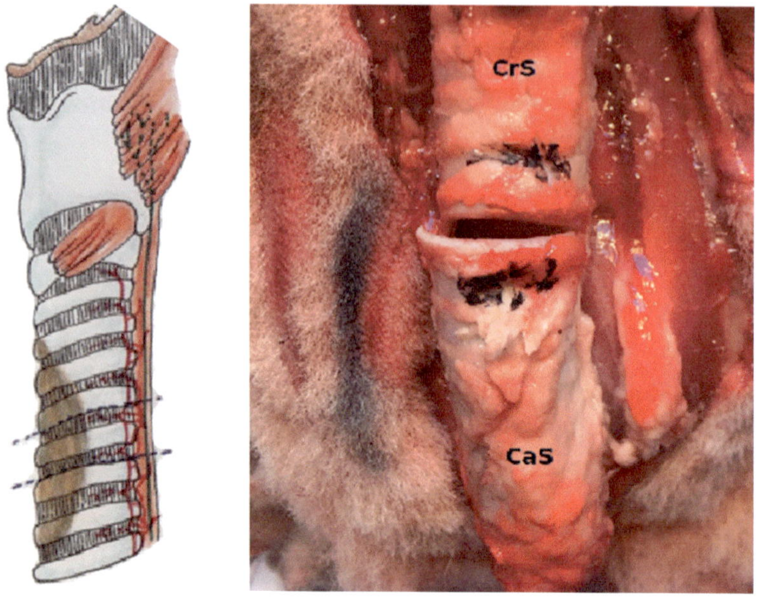

Fig. 5.11 Division of the trachea in the midportion of the stenosis. *CrS* cranial segment of the trachea, *CaS* caudal segment of the trachea

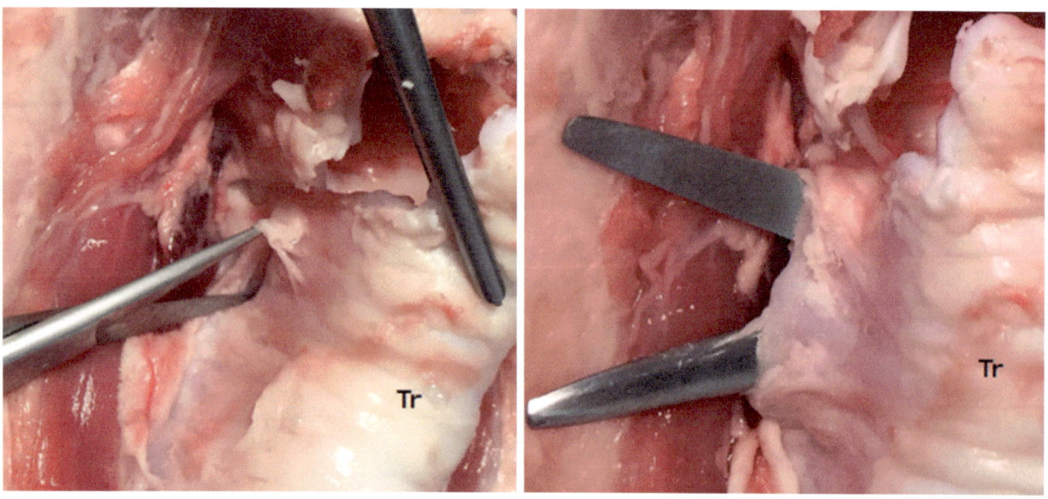

Fig. 5.12 Mobilization of the cranial and caudal segment of the trachea. *Tr* trachea

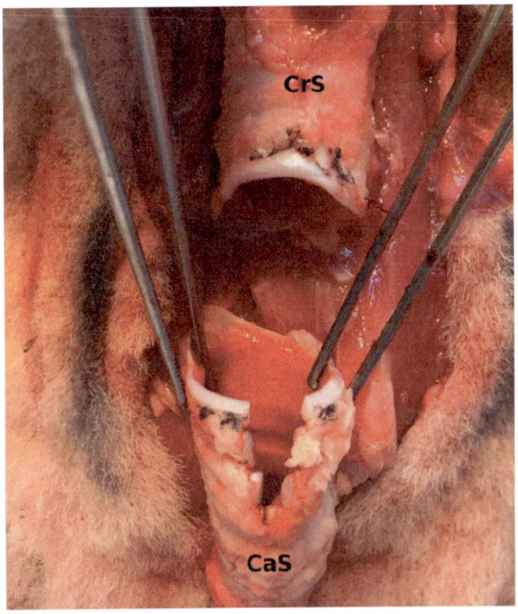

Fig. 5.13 The stenotic segment is longitudinally slit anteriorly on its caudal segment and posteriorly on its cranial segment. *CrS* cranial segment of the trachea, *CaS* caudal segment of the trachea

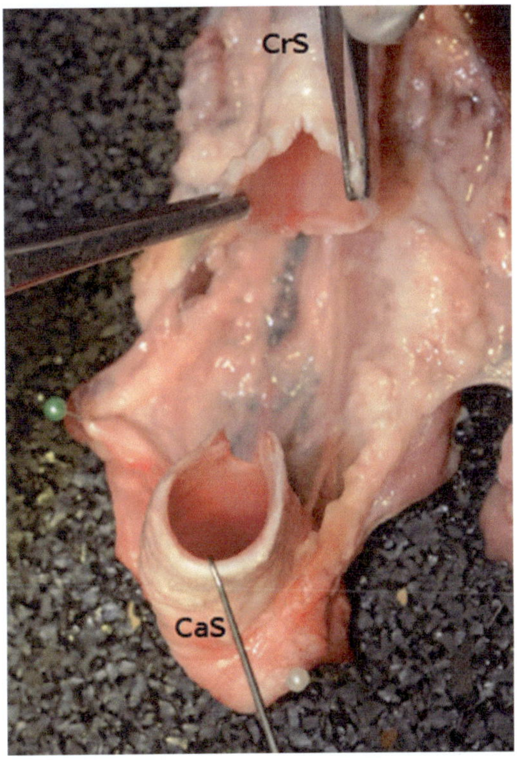

Fig. 5.14 The stenotic segment is longitudinally slit anteriorly on its cranial segment and posteriorly on its caudal segment (Image kindly given by K. Sandu). *CrS* cranial segment of the trachea, *CaS* caudal segment of the trachea

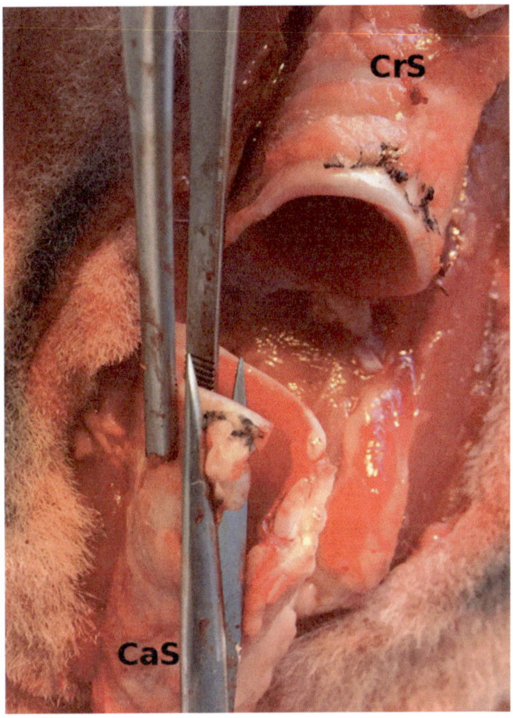

Fig. 5.15 Trimming of the lateral sharp edges of the tracheal stumps. *CrS* cranial segment of the trachea, *CaS* caudal segment of the trachea

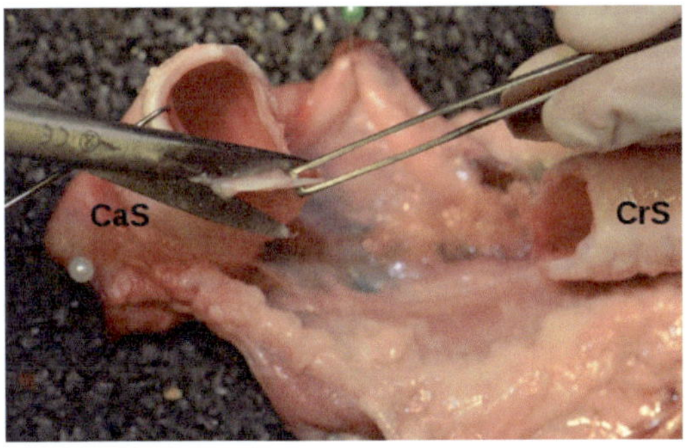

Fig. 5.16 Trimming of the right-angled corners of the tracheal stumps (Image kindly given by K. Sandu). *CrS* cranial segment of the trachea, *CaS* caudal segment of the trachea

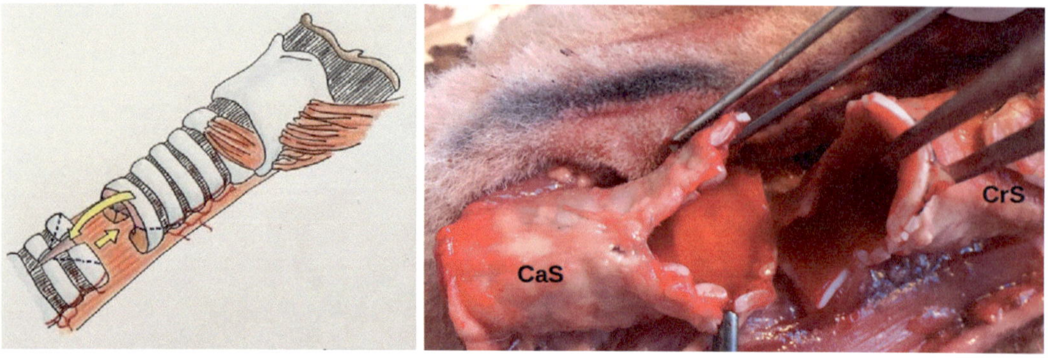

Fig. 5.17 Overlapping of the proximal and distal segment of the trachea, placing the cranial segment anteriorly. *CrS* cranial segment of the trachea, *CaS* caudal segment of the trachea

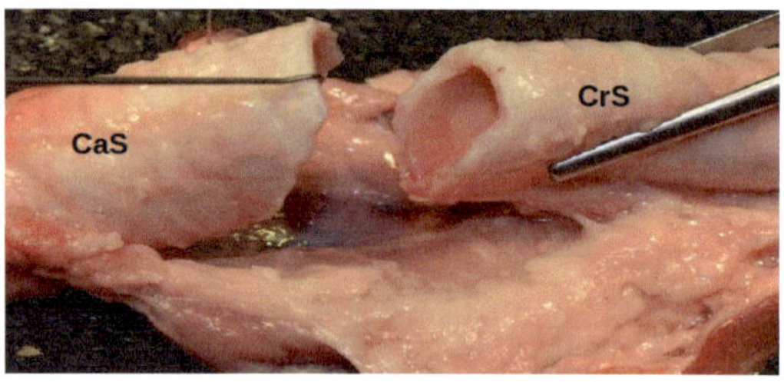

Fig. 5.18 Overlapping of the proximal and distal segment of the trachea, placing the cranial segment posteriorly (Image kindly given by K. Sandu). *CrS* cranial segment of the trachea, *CaS* caudal segment of the trachea

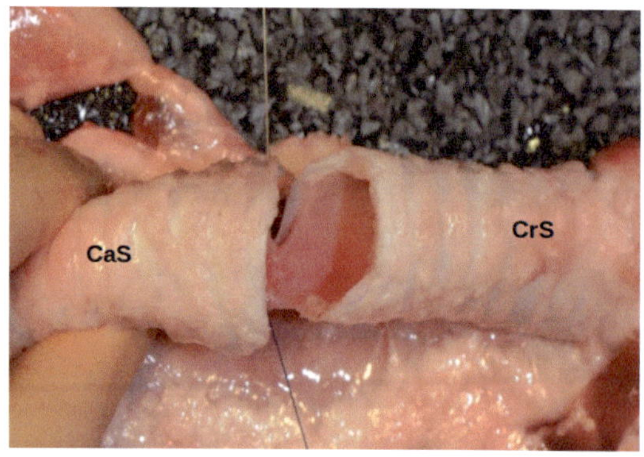

Fig. 5.19 Placing of the first stitch posteriorly (Image kindly given by K. Sandu). *CrS* cranial segment of the trachea, *CaS* caudal segment of the trachea

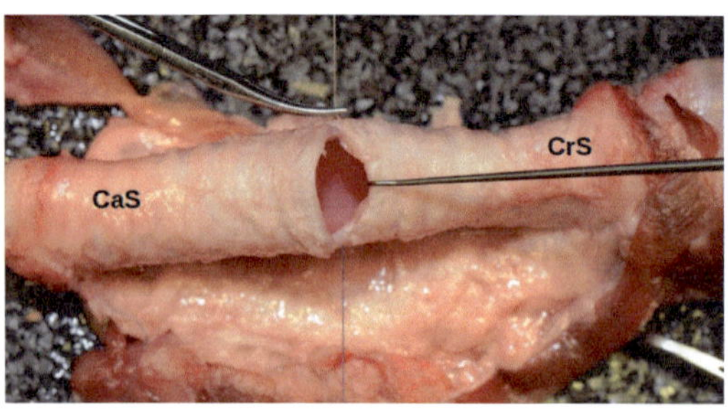

Fig. 5.20 Oblique, oval-shaped anastomosis with two running 4.0 Vicryl sutures from caudal to cranial (Image kindly given by K. Sandu). *CrS* cranial segment of the trachea, *CaS* caudal segment of the trachea

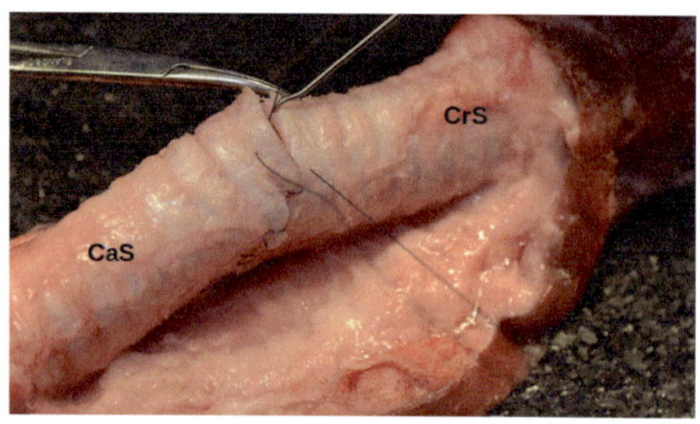

Fig. 5.21 Placing of the last stitches anteriorly (Image kindly given by K. Sandu). *CrS* cranial segment of the trachea, *CaS* caudal segment of the trachea

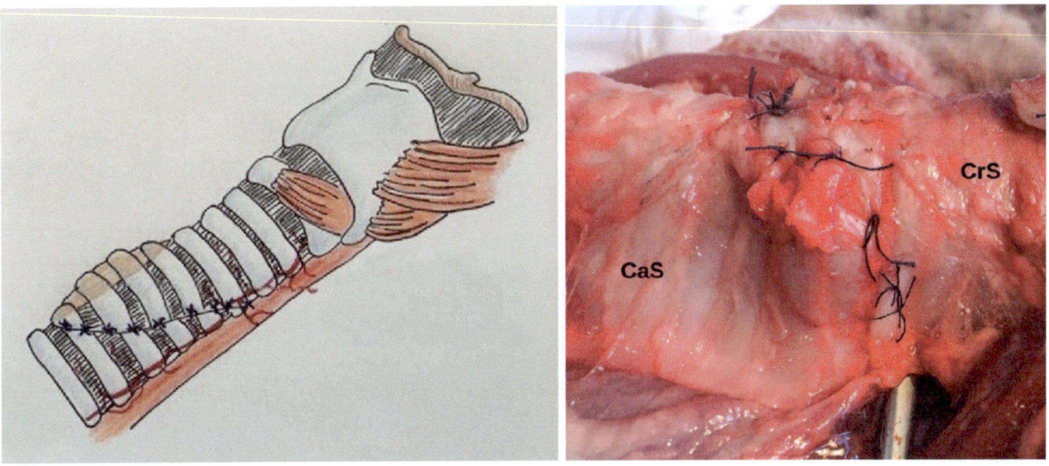

Fig. 5.22 External view of the anastomosis

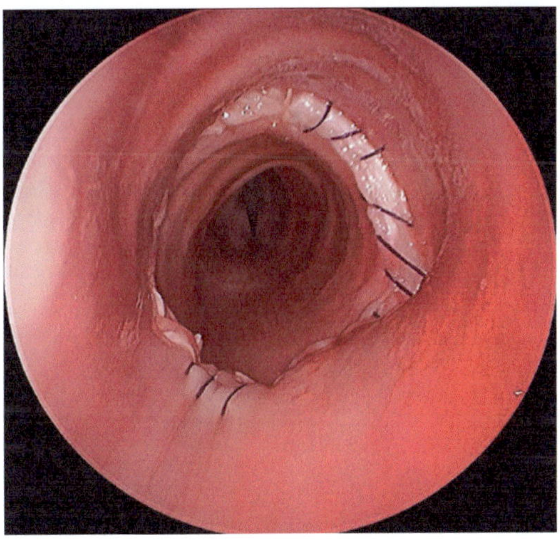

Fig. 5.23 Retrograde endoscopic view of the anastomosis (Image kindly given by K. Sandu)

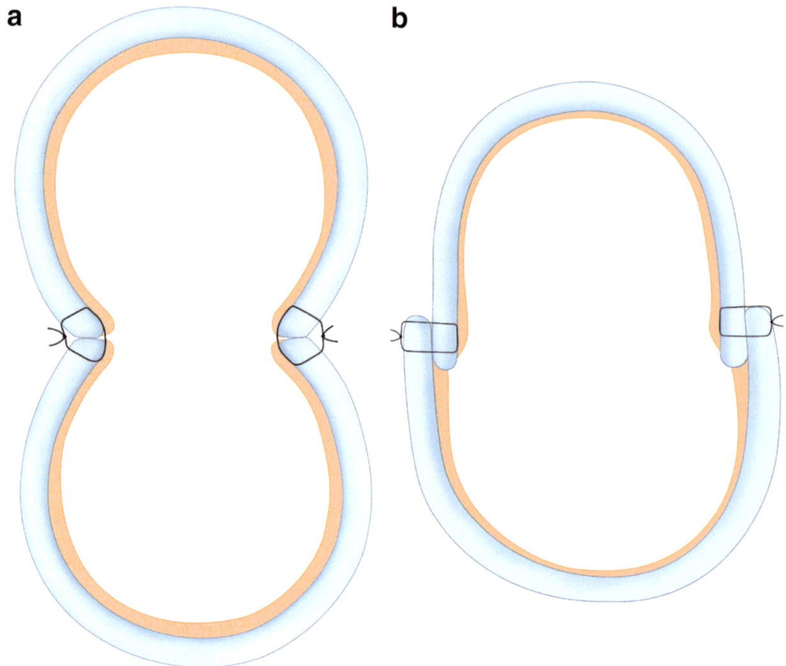

Fig. 5.24 Technical detail of slide tracheoplasty anastomosis: (**a**) when both tracheal stumps are sutured side to side, a figure-eight deformity of the trachea ensues. (**b**) Overlap of the lateral tracheal walls with transfixing mattress sutures prevents the figure-eight deformity from occurring

5.4 Modified Slide Tracheoplasties

Some types of modified slide tracheoplasties are described in humans to treat:

- Dehiscence or restenosis after slide tracheoplasty (secondary reverse slide tracheoplasty [7])
- LSTS involving the carina using an inverted Y-shaped incision in the distal segment [8]
- Upper airway LSTS (latero-lateral slide tracheoplasty [9])
- LSTS in patients with an anomalous right upper lobe bronchus arising separately from the trachea (pig bronchus) [10]

Take-Home Messages

- LSTS is a severe and often life-threatening anatomical anomaly constricting the trachea for >50% of its length.
- Slide tracheoplasty should be the preferred option for the management of LSTS, especially in the young.
- This procedure shortens the trachea by half but doubles its circumference and quadruples its cross-sectional area.
- In slide tracheoplasty, the reconstruction is done with native vascularized cartilaginous trachea, which eliminates malacia and granuloma formation as postoperative complications.

References

1. Gallagher TQ, Hartnick CJ (2012) Slide tracheoplasty. Adv Otorhinolaryngol 73:58–62
2. Butler CR, Speggiorin S, Rijnberg FM, Roebuck DJ, Muthialu N, Hewitt RJ, Elliott MJ (2014) Outcomes of slide tracheoplasty in 101 children: a 17-year single-center experience. J Thorac Cardiovasc Surg 147(6):1783–1789
3. Rutter MJ, Cotton RT, Azizkhan RG, Manning PB (2003) Slide tracheoplasty for the management of complete tracheal rings. J Pediatr Surg 38(6):928–934
4. Macchiarini P, Dulmet E, de Montpreville V, Mazmanian GM, Chapelier A, Dartevelle P (1997) Tracheal growth after slide tracheoplasty. J Thorac Cardiovasc Surg 113(3):558–566
5. Wright CD (2009) Treatment of Congenital Tracheal Stenosis. Semin Thorac Cardiovasc Surg 21(3):274–277
6. Cunningham MJ, Eavey RD, Vlahakes GJ, Grillo HC (1998) Slide tracheoplasty for long-segment tracheal stenosis. Arch Otolaryngol Head Neck Surg 124(1):98–103
7. Kopelovich JC, Wine TM, Rutter MJ, Mitchell MB, Prager JD (2016) Secondary reverse slide tracheoplasty for airway rescue. Ann Thorac Surg 101(3):1205–1207
8. Toma M, Kamagata S, Hirobe S, Komori K, Okumura K, Mutoh M, Hayashi A (2009) Modified slide tracheoplasty for congenital tracheal stenosis. J Pediatr Surg 44(10):2019–2022
9. Tasci E, Ciftci H, Periovi F, Kutlu CA (2009) Latero-lateral slide tracheoplasty for upper airway stenosis: an 8-year follow-up. J Thorac Cardiovasc Surg 137(1):e44–e46
10. Beierlein W, Elliott MJ (2006) Variations in the technique of slide tracheoplasty to repair complex forms of long-segment congenital tracheal stenoses. Ann Thorac Surg 82(4):1540–1542

Step-by-Step Tracheal Resection with End-to-End Anastomosis

6

F. Canzano, E. Aggazzotti Cavazza, F. Mattioli, A. Ghidini, S. Bottero, and L. Presutti

6.1 Introduction

This procedure is a surgical technique for resection of a portion of the trachea followed by end-to-end anastomosis. It is performed in short-segment tracheal stenosis in patients without comorbidities.

Indications for tracheal resection anastomosis were post-intubation stenosis and trauma. One to five tracheal rings were resected.

Tracheal anastomosis is considered successful if the patient remained asymptomatic for 24 months of close follow-up.

Tracheal resection and end-to-end anastomosis are relatively safe and reliable for definitive treatment of benign tracheal stenosis in appropriate patients.

6.2 Surgical Training Step by Step

Step 1 Skin Landmarks Identification and Incision

In order to start the procedure, it is useful to identify main landmarks on the skin; identification by palpation of laryngeal framework in sheep animal model is quite similar to humans.

A horizontal collar incision is made 2 cm above the sternal notch (Fig. 6.1).

Step 3 Superficial Layer Dissection

Elevation of the cutaneous and subplatysmal flaps and identification of the strap muscles.

The strap muscles are divided in the midline by the linea alba.

The stitches are positioned in order to facilitate exposure of the laryngeal framework, the thyroid gland, and the anterior tracheal wall.

F. Canzano (✉) • E. Aggazzotti Cavazza • F. Mattioli
A. Ghidini • S. Bottero • L. Presutti
Head and Neck Department, University Hospital of Modena, Modena, Italy
e-mail: federica.canzano@gmail.com

A. Ghidini et al. (eds.), *Atlas of Airway Surgery*, DOI 10.1007/978-3-319-49739-6_6

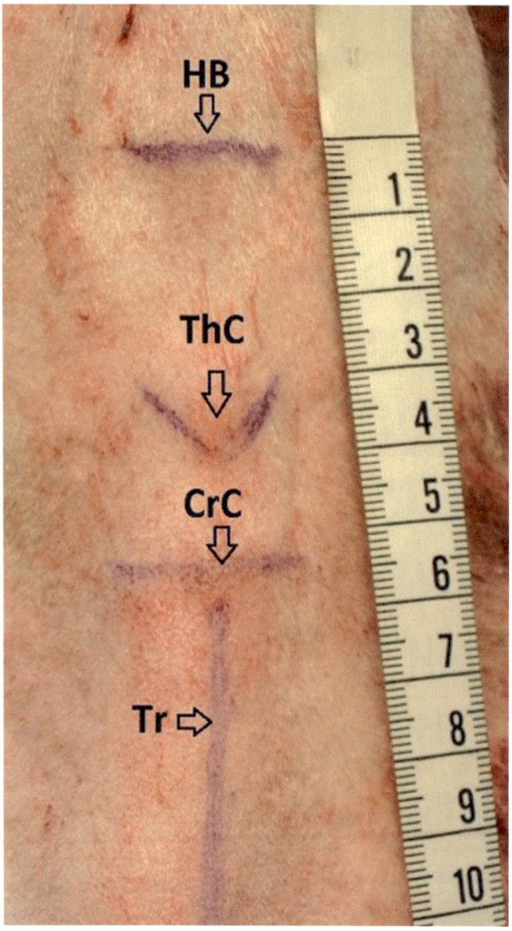

Fig. 6.1 Identification of main landmarks of laryngeal framework

Step 4 Anatomical Study of the Trachea

Below the cricoid cartilage, the surgeon can identify and palpate the first tracheal ring.

Look and study the trachea and identify and palpate any pathologic deformity (Fig. 6.2).

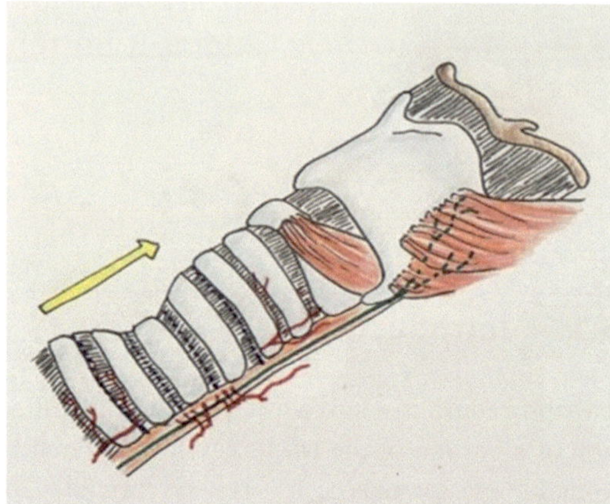

Fig. 6.2 Pathologic tracheal stenosis involving the III, IV and V tracheal rings

Step 5 Mark the Stenosis

Do an intraoperative fibroscopy and identify the exact location of the stenosis.

With the endoscopic light, you can mark with dermographic pen the pathologic tracheal stenosis on anterior tracheal wall (Fig. 6.3).

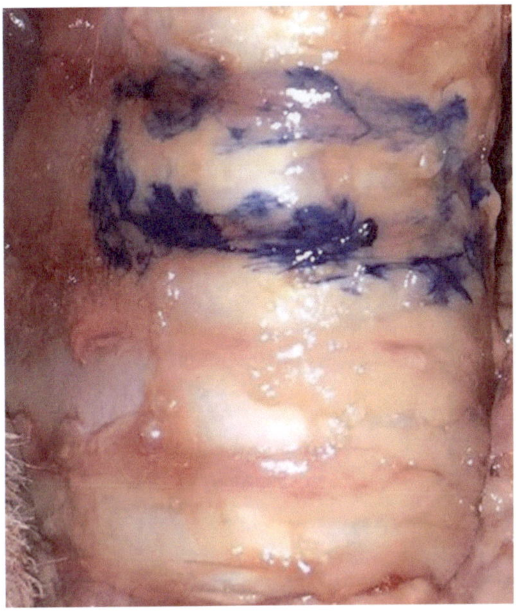

Fig. 6.3 Pen drawing of the pathologic tracheal stenosis

Step 6 Tracheal Dissection

The tracheal dissection is performed by anterolateral direction. The main goals are to mobilize distally the trachea, preserve all the structures located laterally to the trachea, and identify and preserve esophagus. Pay attention to tracheal dissection and remember that all the vascular supply coming bilaterally from the tracheal esophageal groove should be preserved (Fig. 6.4).

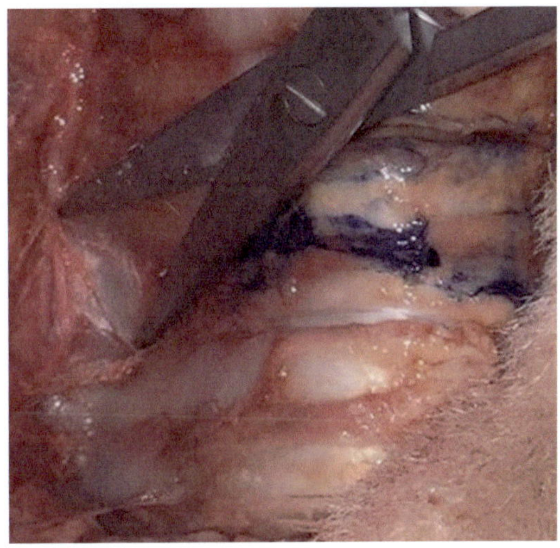

Fig. 6.4 Antero-lateral tracheal dissection

Step 6 Opening of Airways

If exact location of the upper and lower edges of the intrinsic portion of stenosis is identified, it will be best to incise the trachea transversally through the narrowest portion of the airway and progress cranially and caudally until normal tracheal rings are found (Fig. 6.5).

The trachea is opened transversally over and below of the stenosis, which is marked by dermographic pen (Fig. 6.6).

The trachea is then progressively sliced cranially and caudally until normal steady tracheal rings are reached.

During dissection avoid:

- Bipolar coagulation of the feeding vessels to the trachea that could be strictly limited to the stenotic tracheal segment. Feeding vessels to the trachea are only coagulated over the segment that will be resected.
- Circumferential tracheal dissection.

Cut the upper and the lower portion of the trachea.

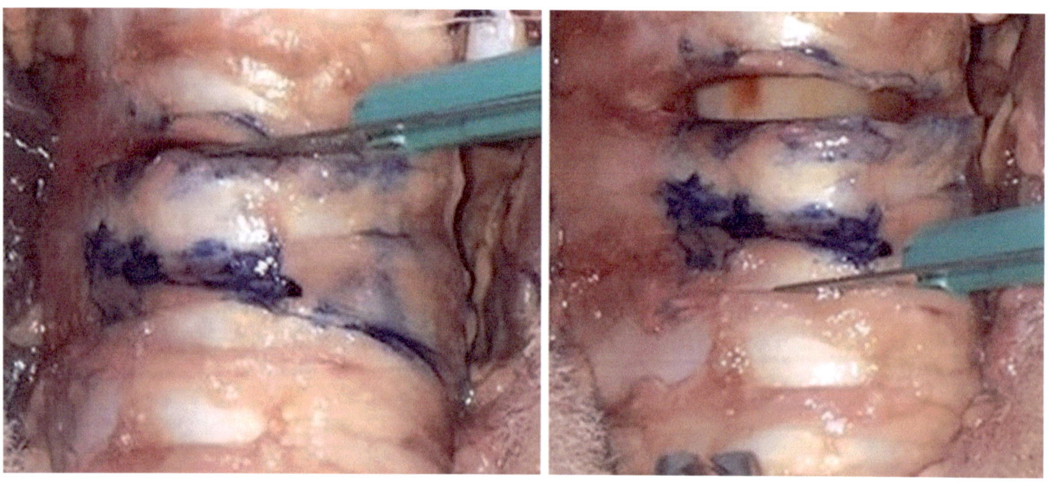

Fig. 6.5 Transversal incision of trachea

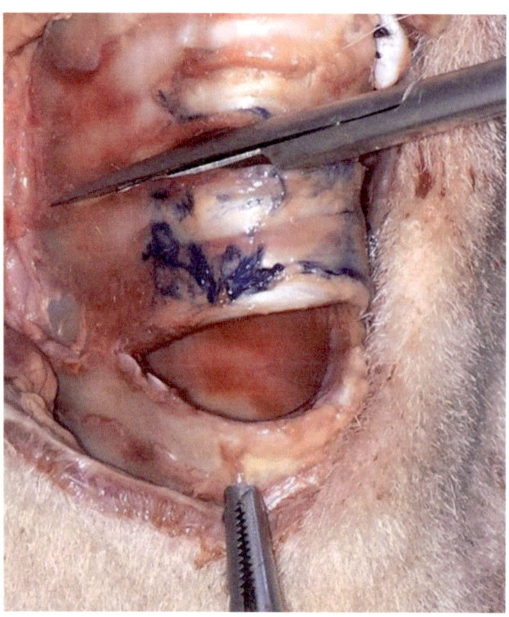

Fig. 6.6 Transversal opening of trachea

Step 8 Posterior Tracheal Dissection
The membranous trachea is dissected and separated from the anterior wall of the esophagus (Figs. 6.7 and 6.8).

Unnecessary extensive separation of the trachea from the esophagus must be avoided in order to preserve an optimal vascular supply to the tracheal stump.

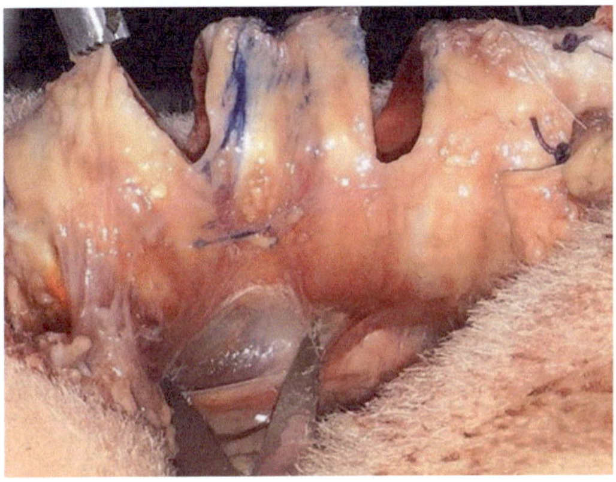

Fig. 6.7 Posterior tracheal dissection

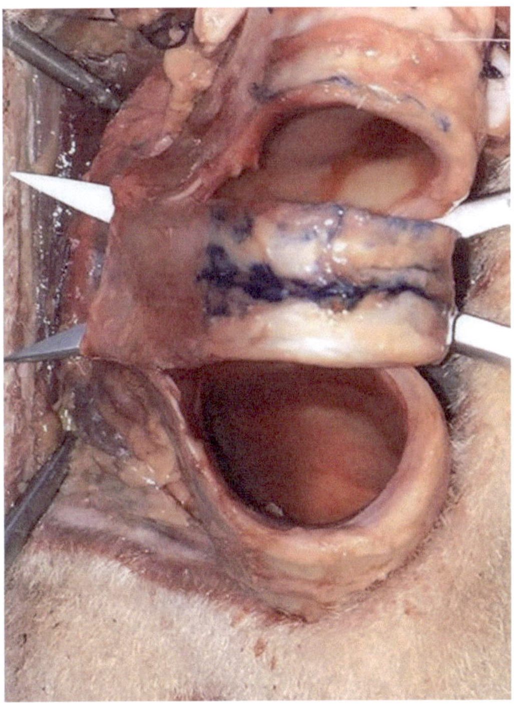

Fig. 6.8 Posterior tracheal dissection

Step 8 Tracheal Resection
Do the tracheal resection with Forbes (Fig. 6.9).

Step 9 Posterior Anastomosis
The proximal and distal stumps of the trachea are usually well matched in performing the anastomosis.

The posterior anastomosis is carried out first. It is done with 3.0 interrupted Vicryl sutures for the membranous trachea. All stitches should emerge in a submucosal plane with the node tied on the outer surface of the trachea (Fig. 6.10).

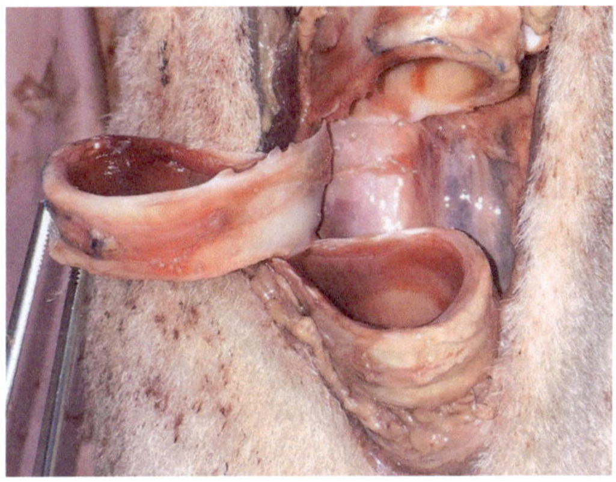

Fig. 6.9 Tracheal resection

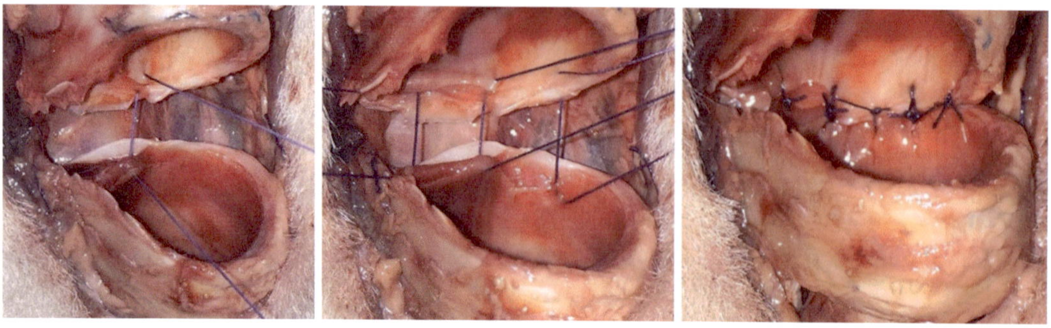

Fig. 6.10 Posterior anastomosis

Step 10 Anterior Anastomosis

The lateral and anterior anastomosis is then performed with interrupted 2.0 Vicryl stitches (Fig. 6.11).

The strap muscles are resutured at the midline, and the skin is closed in two layers. All stitches are placed keeping the needle in a submucosal plane throughout the length of the transcartilaginous stitch, thus avoiding devascularization of the mucosa at the site of anastomosis (Fig. 6.12).

If these basic principles explained in this training step-by-step dissection were respected by all surgeons, the outcome of surgery for tracheal stenosis would certainly be much better.

Improved medical and resident education is of key importance in this field.

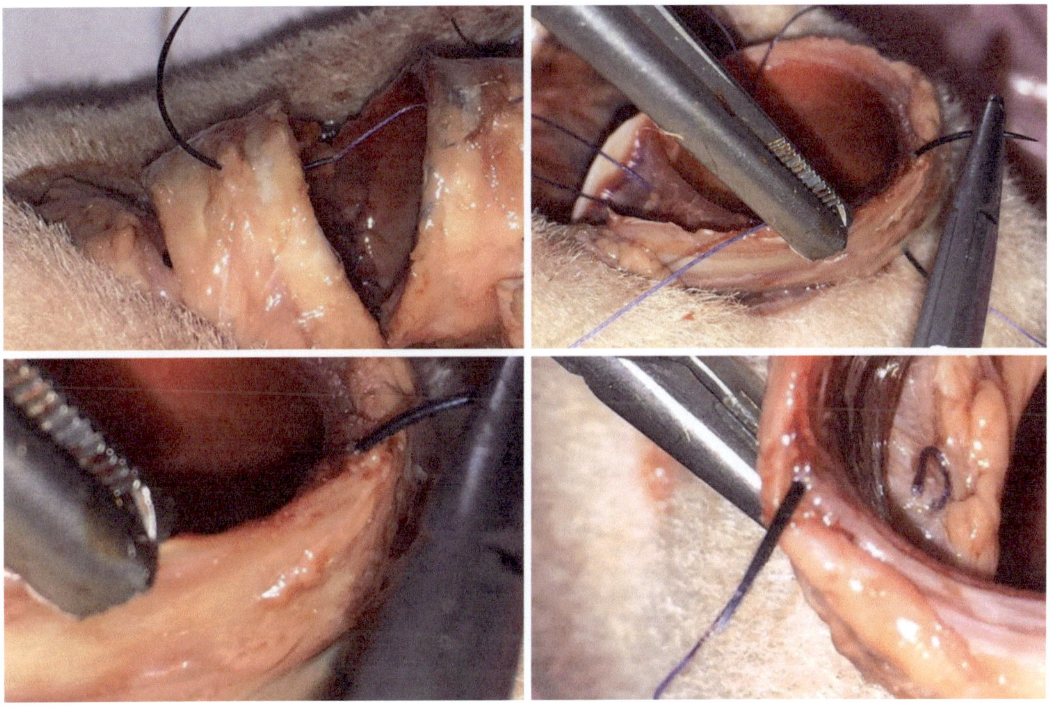

Fig. 6.11 Suture with stiches done in a submucosal plane

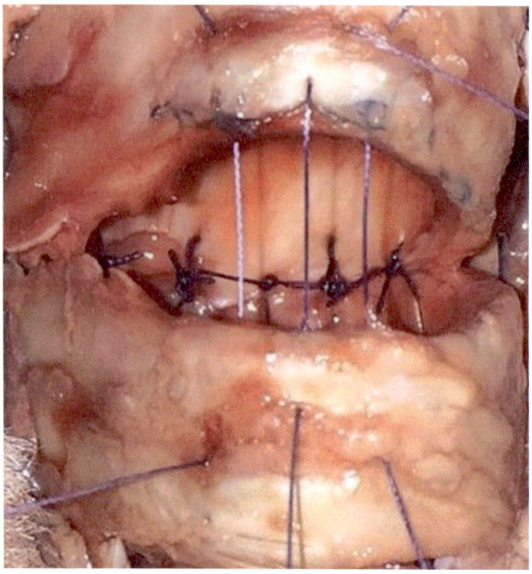

Fig. 6.12 Anterior anastomosis

7 Step-by-Step Partial Cricotracheal Resection (PCTR)

M. Ghirelli, E. Aggazzotti Cavazza, F. Mattioli, A. Ghidini, S. Bottero, and L. Presutti

7.1 Introduction

The first description of partial cricotracheal resection with preservation of the posterior cricoid plate and recurrent laryngeal nerves (RNLs) was made in 1974 by Gerwat and Bryce [1].

PCTR procedure is performed in isolated severe laryngotracheal stenosis (Grade III or IV SGS) in patients without comorbidities.

The concept of removing the diseased airway segment has developed into an attractive alternative to cartilage expansion of the subglottic airway. PCTR with primary thyrotracheal anastomosis spares the glottis with reconstruction of a "normal," rounded, mucosalized subglottic airway.

In 1975 Pearson et al. introduced the technique of transverse resection of the subglottic airway [2].

Lausanne experience involving 15 cases [3] in 1993, with further updates of 100 cases in 2009 [4], showed PCTR is alternative to LTR for selective pediatric cases.

Over the last two decades, PCTR has been advocated as a superior alternative to LTR for the cure of severe Grades III and IV SGS by several authors [3–6].

7.2 Instrumentation and Equipment

If possible, it is better to work in pairs.

Before starting your laboratory session, you should have these materials on hand (Fig. 7.1):

- Dissection tray or a diaper
- Dissection tools: scalpel N°15 and 11 (a); needle driver (b); surgical and anatomic forceps (c); small curved mosquito forceps (d); Kocher's forceps (e); Mayo, curved, and straight iris scissors (f); suture threads 1,0, 2-0, 3-0, and 4-0 (g); Killian's speculum (h); small retractors (i); and a suction cannula (j)
- Medical gauzes (k)
- Paper towel

M. Ghirelli (✉) • E. Aggazzotti Cavazza • F. Mattioli
A. Ghidini • L. Presutti
Head and Neck Department, University Hospital of Modena, Modena, Italy
e-mail: michael.ghirelli@gmail.com

S. Bottero
Airway Surgery Unit, Laryngotracheal Team Director, Bambino Gesù Children's Hospital, Rome, Italy

A. Ghidini et al. (eds.), *Atlas of Airway Surgery*, DOI 10.1007/978-3-319-49739-6_7

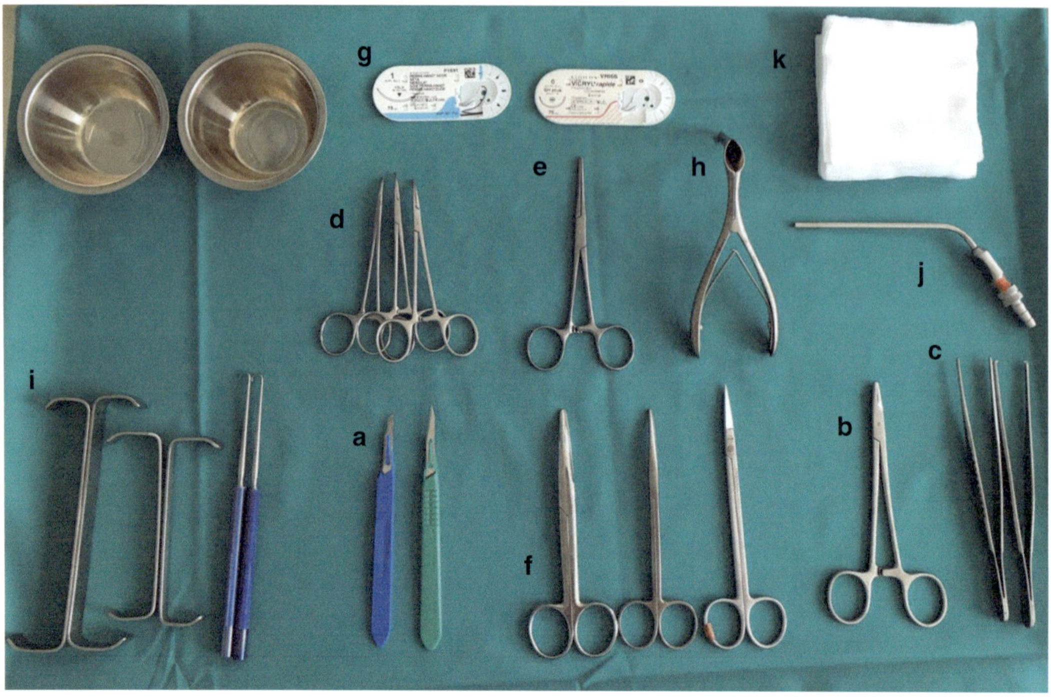

Fig. 7.1 (**a**) Scalpel N°15 and 11, (**b**) needle driver, (**c**) surgical and anatomic forceps, (**d**) small curved mosquito forceps, (**e**) Kocher's forceps, (**f**) Mayo, curved, and straight iris scissors, (**g**) suture threads 1, 0, 2–0, 3–0, 4–0, (**h**) Killian's speculum, (**i**) small retractors, and (**j**) a suction cannula

7.3 Surgical Training Step-by-Step

Step 1 Skin Landmark Identification
Recognition of the main landmarks on the skin (Fig. 7.2) is probably the most simple and fundamental step in all surgical head and neck procedures. Identification by palpation of laryngeal framework in sheep animal model is quite similar to human. In order to start the procedure, it is useful to identify superficial landmarks (Fig. 7.2):

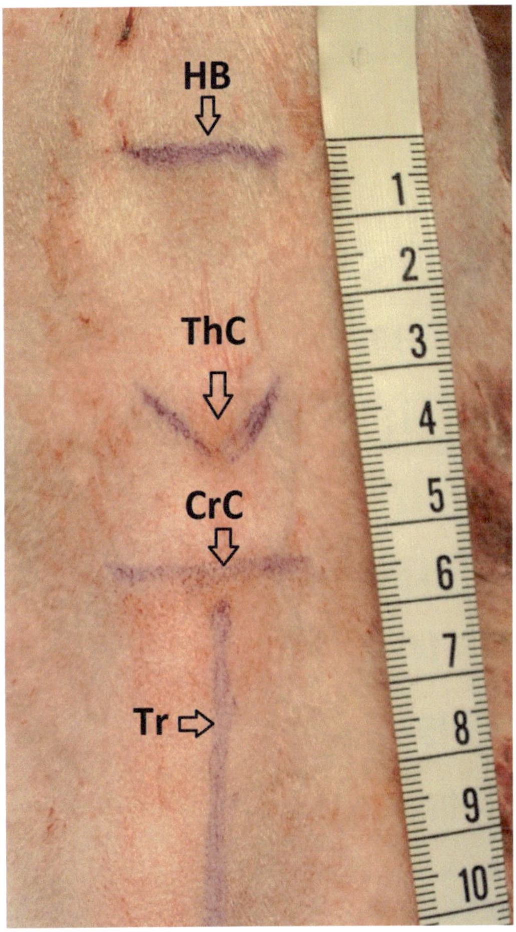

Fig. 7.2 Superficial landmark identification. *HB* hyoid bone, atrial cover by the muscles, *ThC* thyroid cartilage, *Cr* cricoid cartilage, *Tr* trachea

Step 2 Superficial Layer Dissection
Make a vertical incision about 13 cm in order to show the superficial fascia that covers muscles of the neck (Fig. 7.3). Incision could be performed with 10 or 15 blades.

In this step, the main goal is to elevate only a cutaneous and subcutaneous flap.

When all superficial fascia is exposed, the surgeon has to dissect it on the midline with surgical scissor or blade. After this, to allow a good exposition of the main structures below is useful to suture subcutaneous tissue at the lateral skin in its upper and lower part (Fig. 7.3).

Step 3 Laryngeal Framework Identification
When the dissection of the superficial layers is completed, it is important to identify the main structures of laryngeal framework and muscles surrounding it (Fig. 7.4).

The anatomic difference between human and sheep is well described in anatomical chapter. Our goal is to perform a correct dissection plane by plane in order to respect and identify the structures.

Step 4 Infrahyoid Muscle Dissection
Infrahyoid muscles are retracted laterally, resulting in optimal exposure of the lower edge of the thyroid cartilage over its entire width.

It is useful to suture the bigger muscles to subcutaneous layer in order to maintain a wide surgical field. This step simulates the strap muscle dissection on the midline performed in the human procedure in order to expose the hyoid bone and trachea. Sheep thyroid has not an isthmus, so it is not necessary to split the thyroid gland on the midline (Fig. 7.5a).

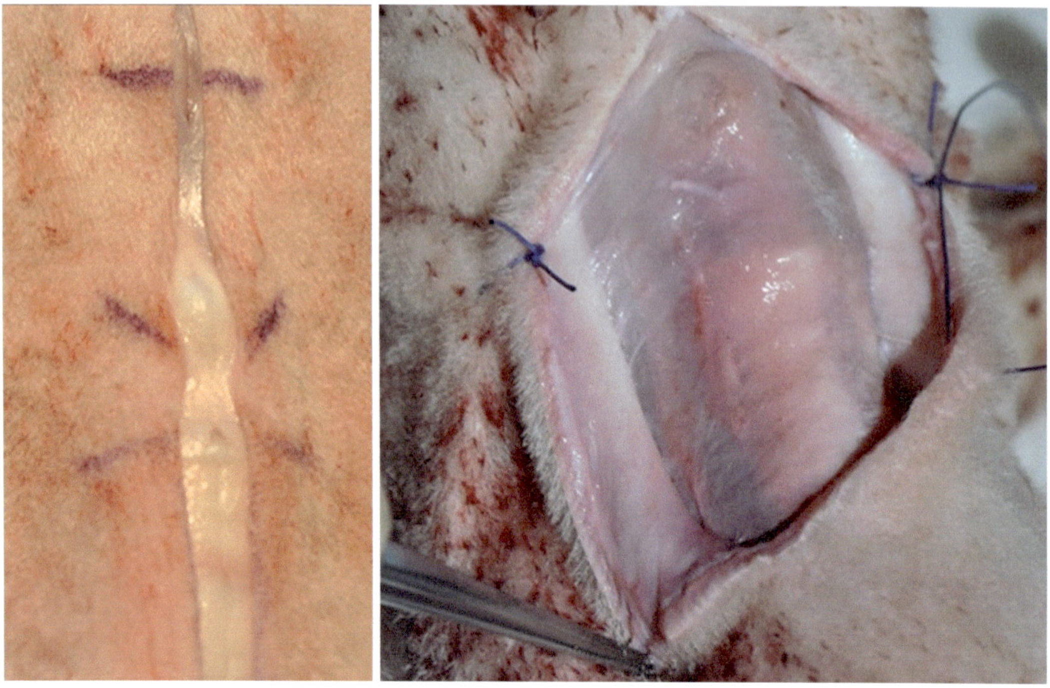

Fig. 7.3 Skin incision. Superficial cervical fascia dissected and sutured with subcutaneous tissue. Below laryngeal's structures covered by its fascia

Now, it is possible to identify all the landmarks (Fig. 7.5b):

- *MyH*: mylohyoid muscle
- *StH*: sternohyoid muscle
- *CrM*: cricothyroid muscles
- *ThH*: thyrohyoid muscles
- *StM*: sternothyroid muscle
- *ThC*: thyroid cartilage
- *Cr*: cricoid cartilage
- *Tr*: trachea
- *Thy*: thyroid gland

Step 5 Dissection of the Trachea

The dissection of the trachea (Fig. 7.6) is done only anteriorly and slightly laterally without identifying the recurrent laryngeal nerves (RNLs). Surgical pearls to avoid RNLs injury are:

- Stay close contact with the outer perichondrium of the tracheal rings.
- RLN identification on sheep animal model is not the goal of procedure. In human procedure to minimize RLN injury, dissection must be carried out against the trachea without recurrent laryngeal nerve visualization.
- Avoid dissection above the posterolateral border of the cricoid plate in order to avoid injury to the RLNs.

The vascular supply of the trachea is into the tracheoesophageal groove, and it must be preserved. On animal model, optimal hemostasis over the tracheal segment that is to be resected is not possible, but this step is crucial to reduce risk of RLN injury.

Step 6 Opening of Airways

Dissect and reflect the cricothyroid muscles over the cricothyroid joints by sharp dissection off the cricoid ring from the midline so as to protect the RLNs (Fig. 7.7a and b).

Open the airway first at the superior edge of the cricoid. Perform the upper resection line along the inferior edge of the thyroid cartilage and stay anterior to the cricothyroid joint, laterally, in order

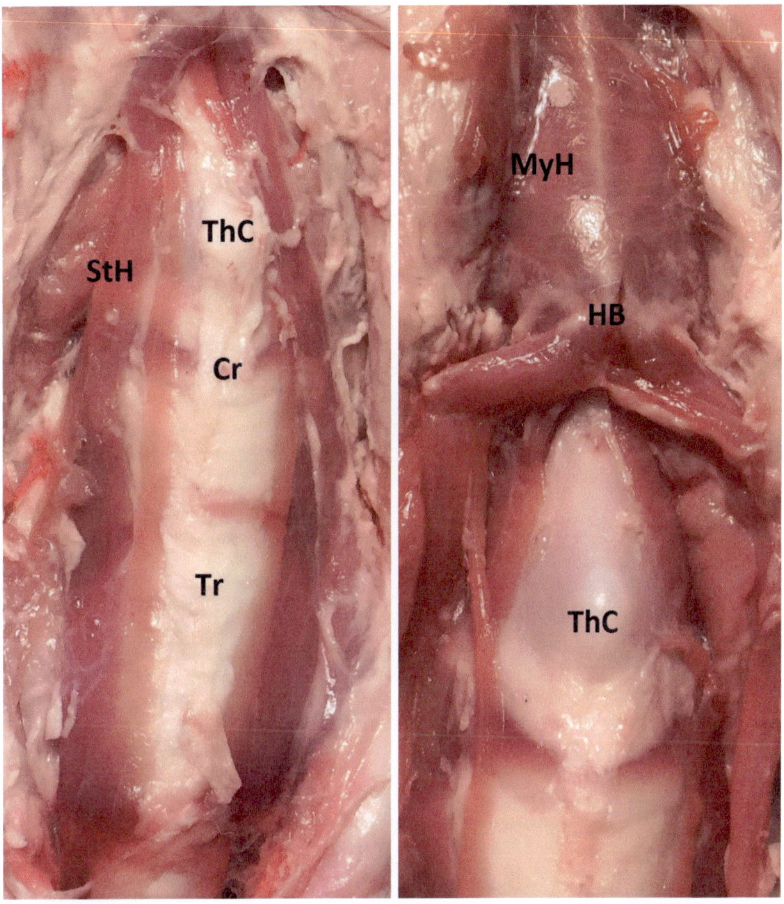

Fig. 7.4 The larynx exposed with muscles surrounding it. *MyH* mylohyoid muscle; *HB* hyoid bone, partial cover by the muscles; *StH* sternohyoid muscle, *ThC* thyroid cartilage, *Cr* cricoid cartilage, *Tr* trachea

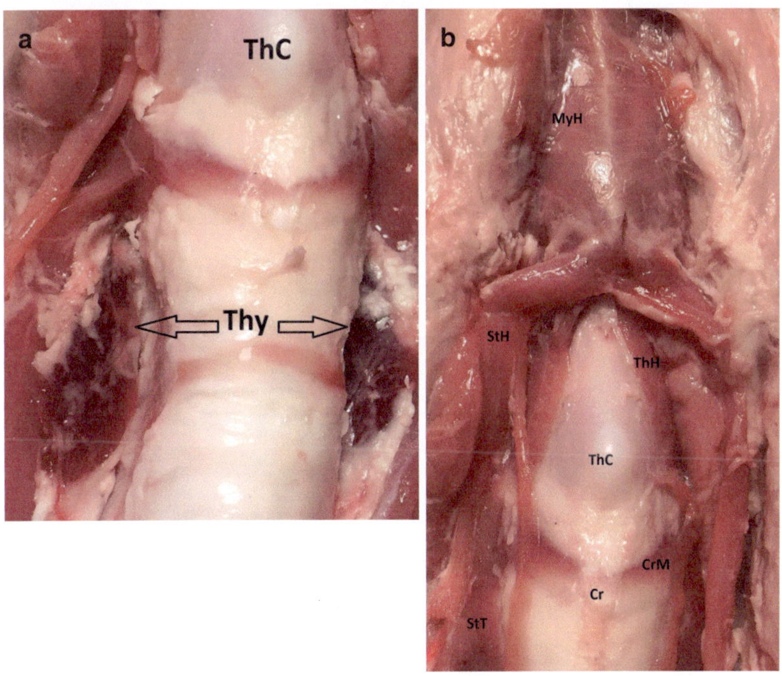

Fig. 7.5 (**a**) Strap muscles dissected and mylohyoid muscle. (**b**) Thyroid gland dissected and trachea

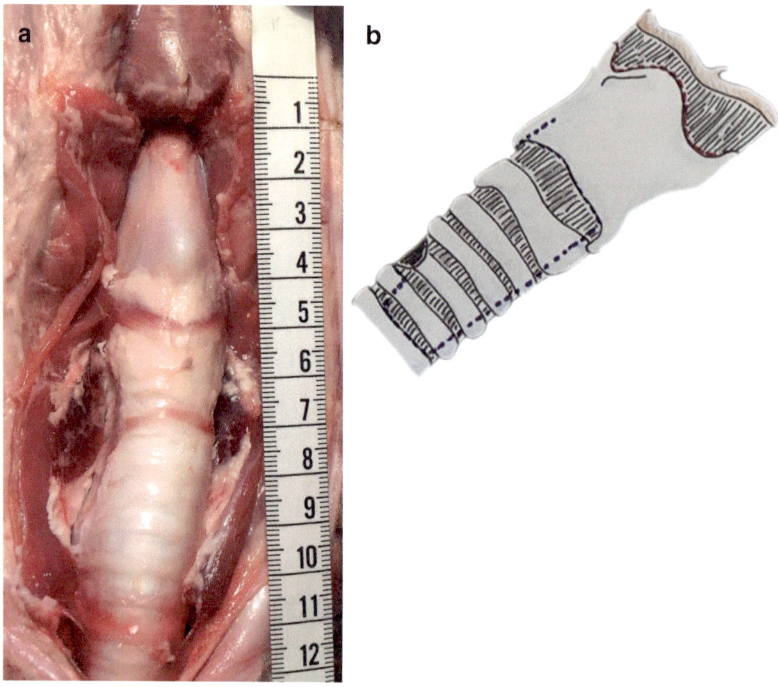

Fig. 7.6 (**a**) Exposure of tracheal laryngeal axis. (**b**) The resection lines (*dotted blue lines*) for partial cricotracheal resection

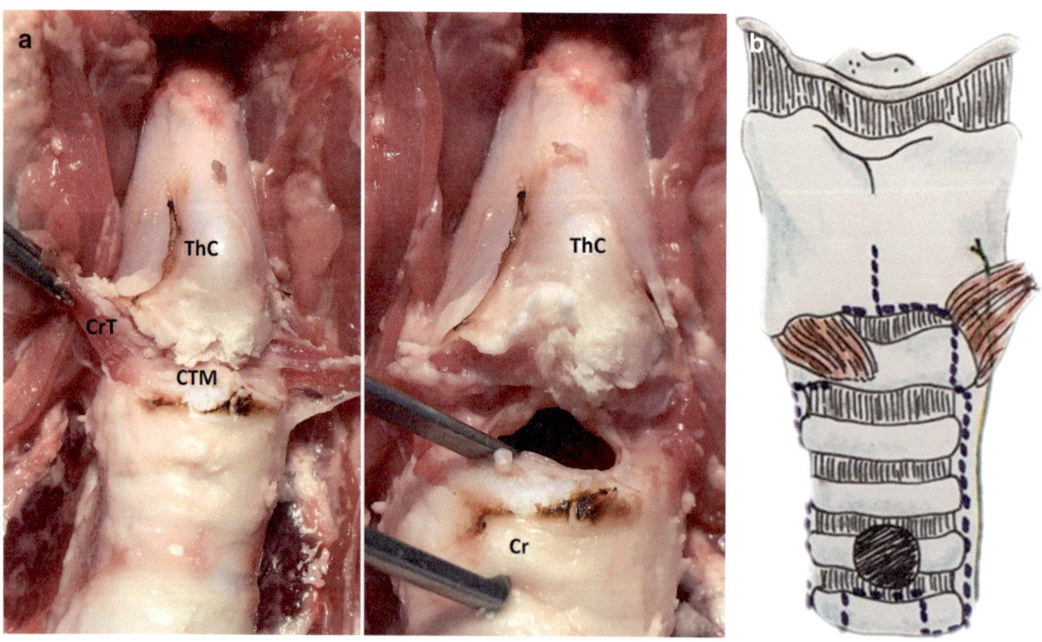

Fig. 7.7 (**a**) Airway opened at cricothyroid membrane after cricothyroid muscle dissection. (**b**) Cricothyroid muscles reflected in order to protect RLN

to avoid injury to the RLNs. Once the skeleton of the anterior cricoid arch has been freed, a view of the posterior cricoid plate is obtained through the former cricothyroid membrane:

- *CTM:* cricothyroid membrane
- *ThH*: cricothyroid muscles
- *ThC*: thyroid cartilage
- *Cr*: cricoid cartilage

Step 7 Subglottic Mucosa Incision

Under visual control, the posterior subglottic mucosa is incised transversally just above the upper limit of the potential stenosis (Fig. 7.8); the mucosa is reflected downward in its subperichondrial layer to expose the posterior cricoid cartilage (Fig. 7.9).

Step 8 Trachea Dissection and Cricotracheal Resection

The membranous trachea is dissected and separated from the anterior wall of the esophagus. This dissection is extended caudally to the level for single-stage PCTR. Unnecessary extensive separation of the trachea from the esophagus must be avoided in order to preserve an optimal vascular supply to the tracheal stump (Figs. 7.10 and 7.11).

When the tracheal dissection is completed, is possible to make the resection of the cricoid cartilage and trachea rings involved by subglottic stenosis (Fig. 7.12).

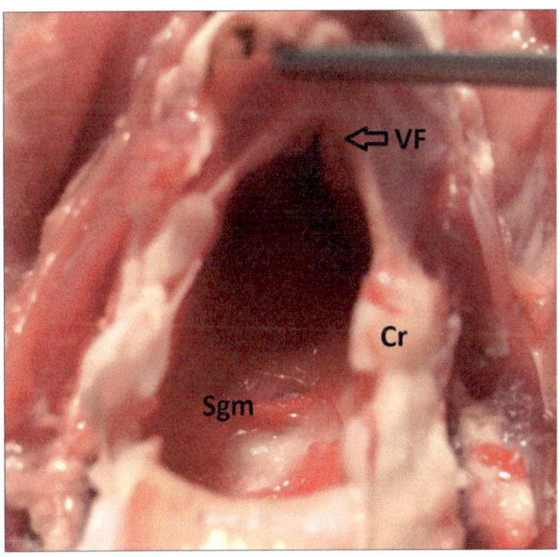

Fig. 7.8 *VF* vocal fold, *Cr* cricoid cartilage, *Sgm* subglottic mucosa

Step 9 Posterior Cricotracheal Anastomosis

Interrupted suture has to be performed with Vicryl 5.0-6.0.

The three posterior stitches are placed at full thickness through the mucosa of the tracheal side and at half thickness through the posterior cricoid plate and subglottic mucosa to achieve perfect mucosal approximation (Fig. 7.13a, b, c).

The posterolateral stitches are passed through the tracheal posterolateral mucosa and the cricoid plate where they must emerge in a subperichondrial plane on the outer surface in order to avoid injury to the recurrent laryngeal nerves (Figs. 7.13d and 7.14).

The knots of the posterior anastomosis are tied inside the lumen, after having pulled the trachea cranially with traction sutures to avoid undue tension on the more fragile posterior anastomosis. All stitches are placed before they are tied inside the lumen. A Vicryl thread does not cause granulation tissue formation, which is usually due to a defective anastomosis technique with inappropriate mucosal approximation (Fig. 7.15).

Step 10 Anterior Cricotracheal Anastomosis

The thyrotracheal anastomosis is completed by placing *3-0, 4-0 Vicryl* sutures between the subglottic thyroid cartilage and the first and second tracheal rings in alternate fashion. Staying in a subperichondrial plane at the cricoid level is essential to avoid injury to the recurrent laryngeal nerves (Fig. 7.16).

Next, a tension-releasing suture is placed through the third or fourth tracheal ring laterally and through the lateral aspect of thyroid cartilage (Fig. 7.17).

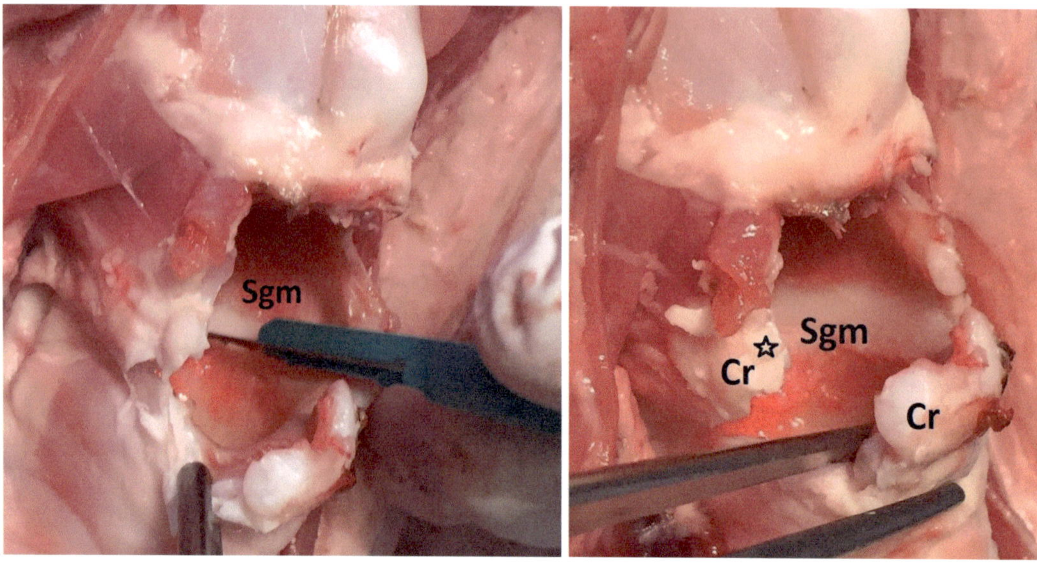

Fig. 7.9 *Sgm* incision of subglottic mucosa, *Cr* cricoid cartilage dissected and posterior part of cricoid cartilage (*star*)

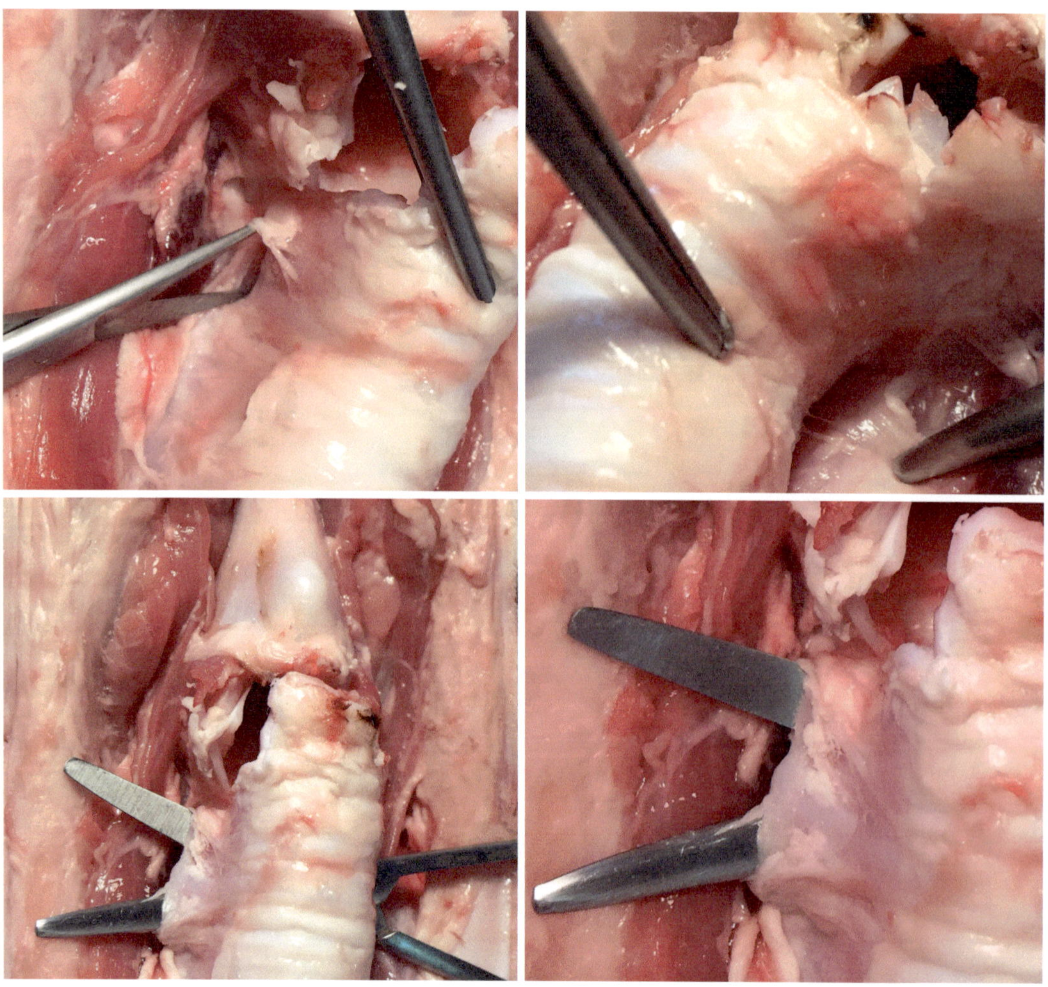

Fig. 7.10 Tracheal dissection with surgical scissor. Pictures show how to stay close to trachea during dissection

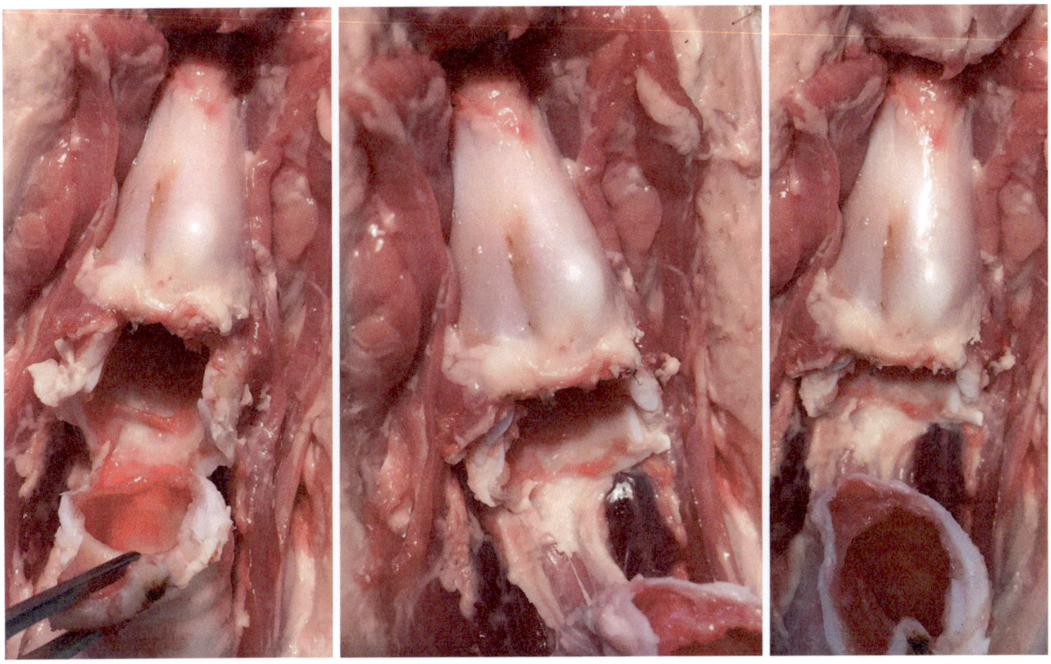

Fig. 7.11 Dissection and removal of subglottic mucosa in order to avoid cicatricial stenosis

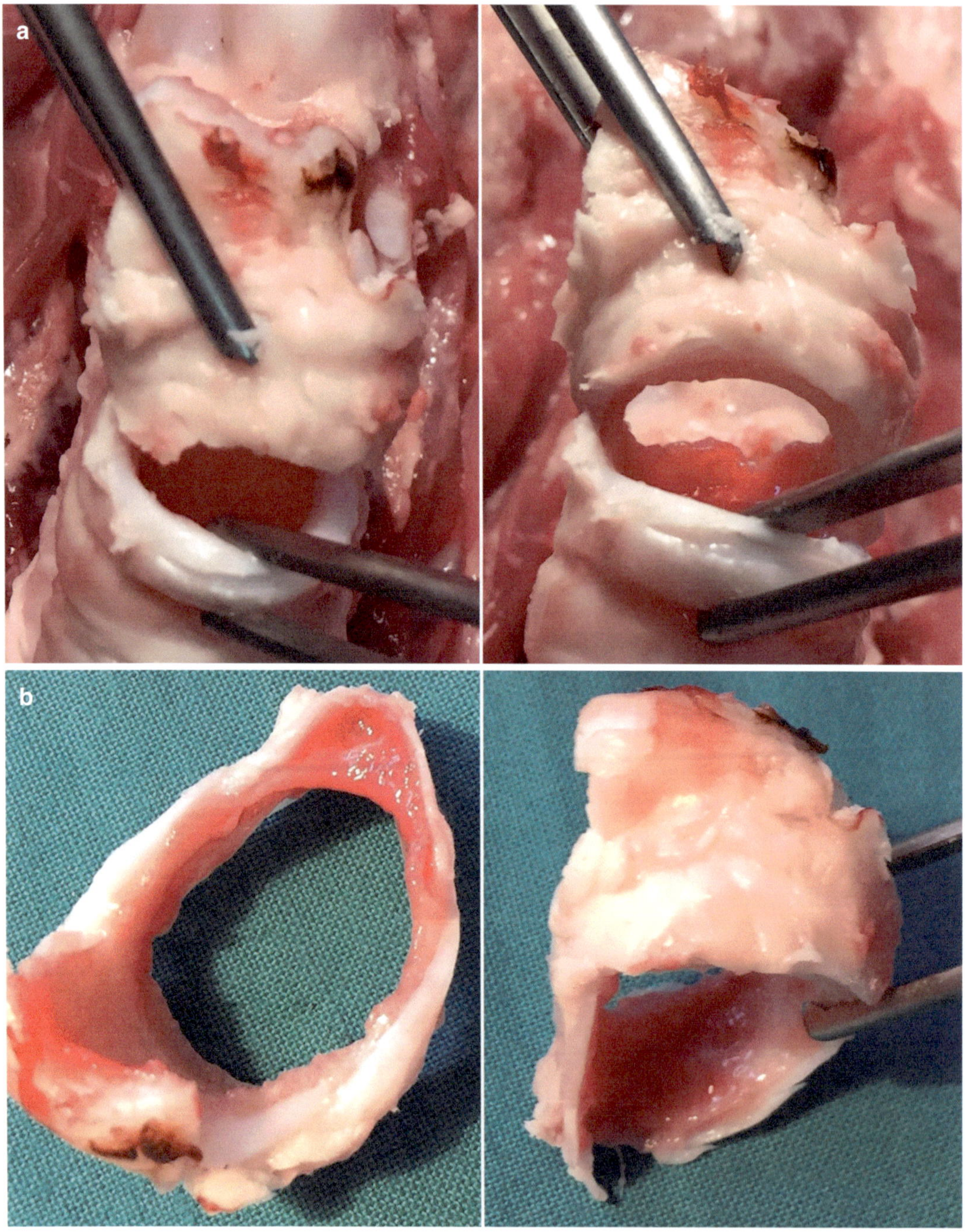

Fig. 7.12 (**a**) Stenotic segment resection and (**b**) cricoid cartilage and trachea's rings

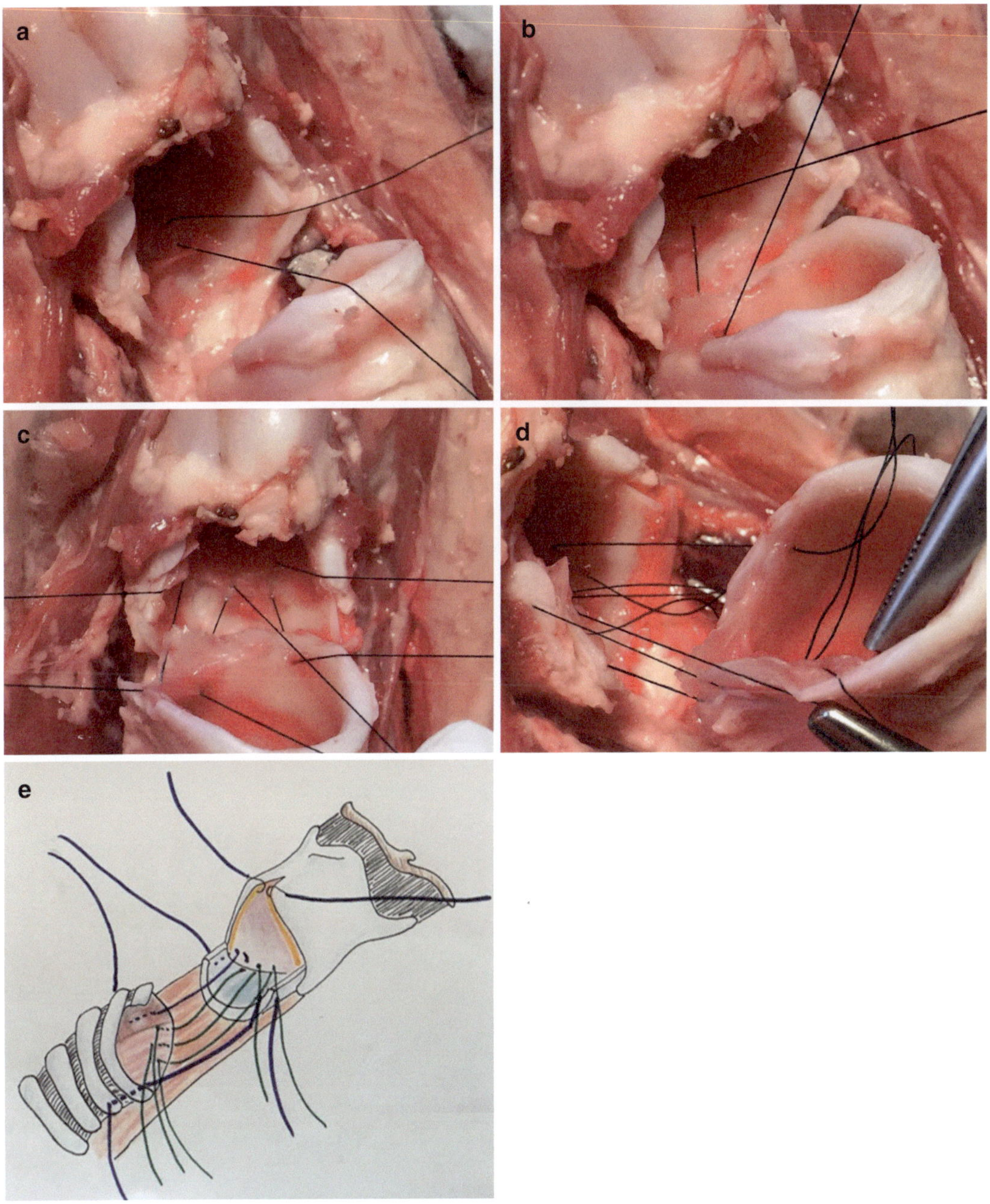

Fig. 7.13 (a–e) Posterior and posterolateral stitches positioning

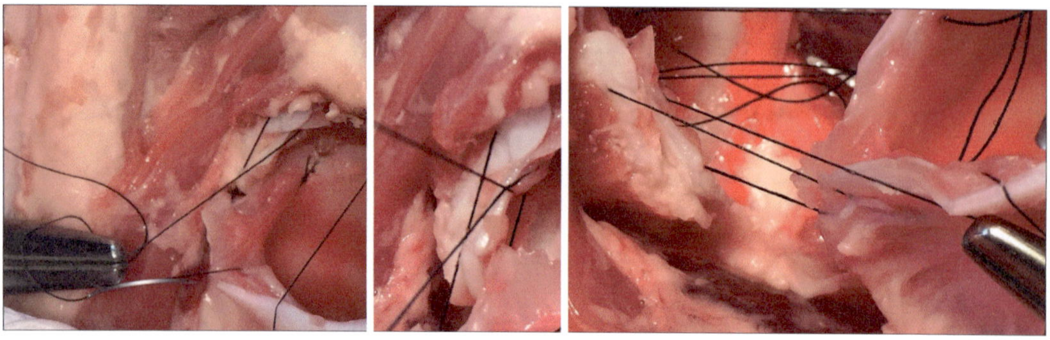

Fig. 7.14 Posterolateral stitch is essential to preserve RLNs and achieve a perfect approximation of the subglottic and trachea mucosae

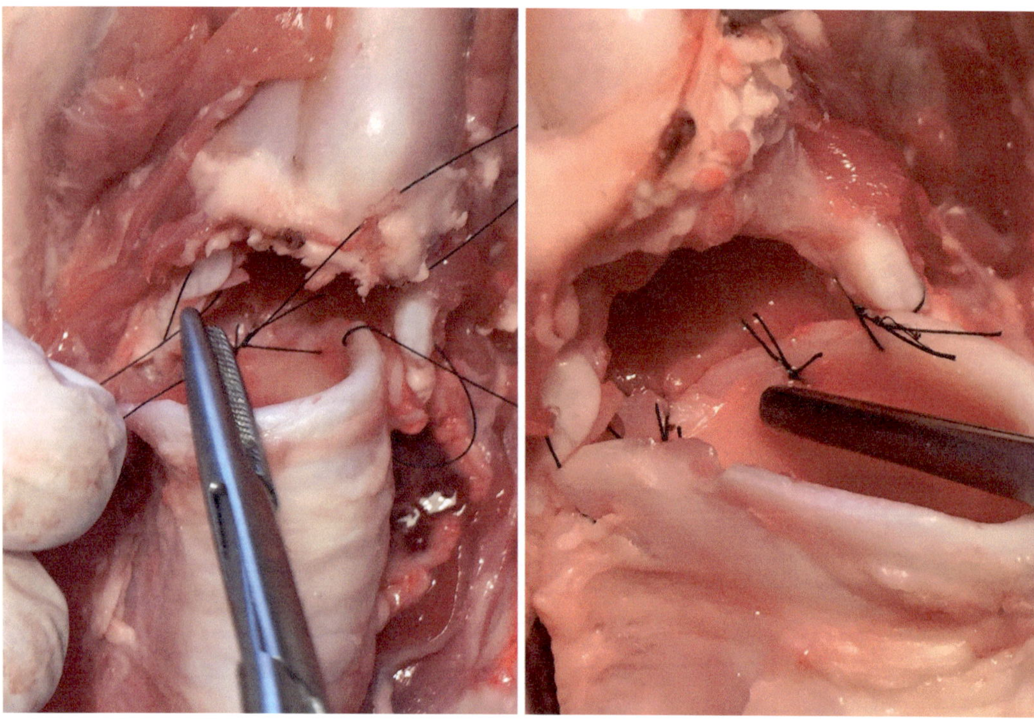

Fig. 7.15 Posterior cricotracheal anastomosis ended

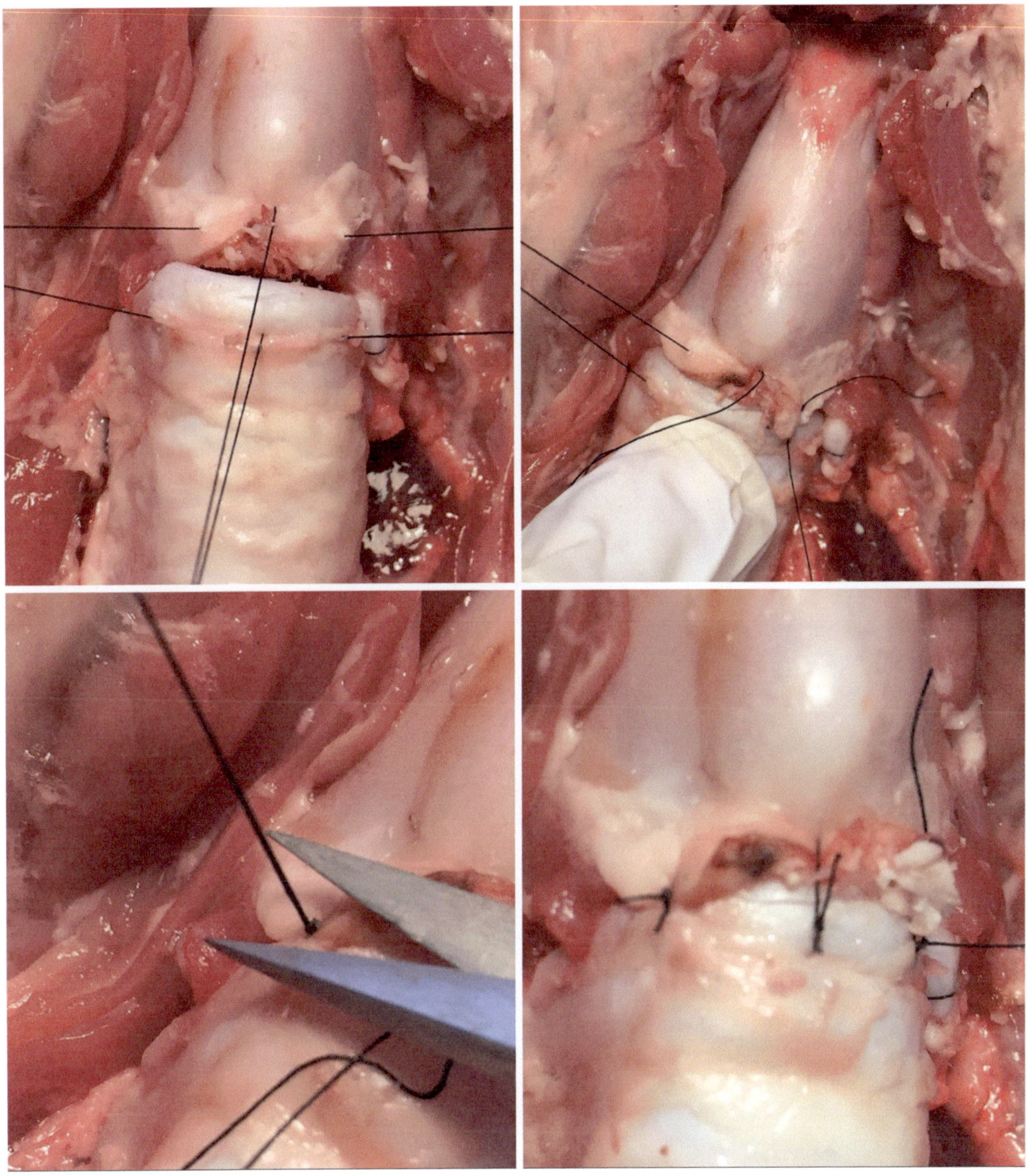

Fig. 7.16 Anterior stitches positioned between the trachea and thyroid cartilage

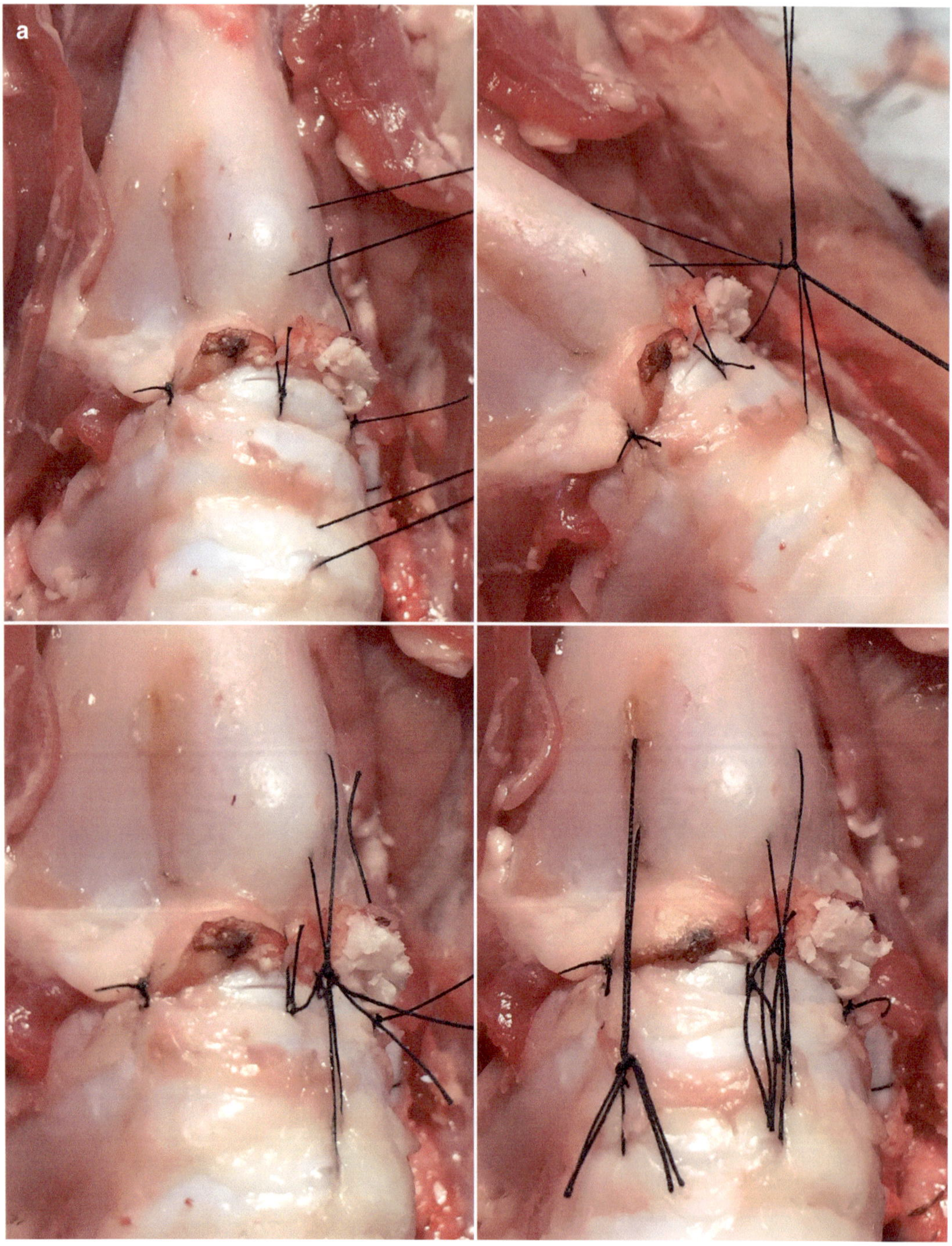

Fig. 7.17 (**a**, **b**) Final anterior stitches in order to stabilize the anastomosis

b

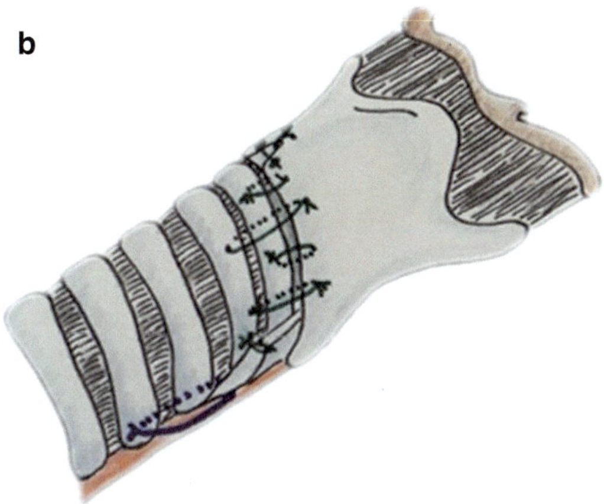

Fig. 7.17 (continued)

Take-Home Message

During training, step-by-step dissection and meticulous respect for all anatomic landmarks are the best way to improve surgical technique.

Similar to human procedure, identification of RLNs is not required.

Cricothyroid muscles reflect over the cricothyroid joint, and subperichondrial tracheal dissection is mandatory to avoid RLN injury.

Stitches positioning in particular the posterolateral ones is a core step to perform a perfect anastomosis.

Perfect mucosal approximation during anastomosis is fundamental to reduce risk of subsequent restenosis.

References

1. Gerwat J, Bryce DP (1974) Management of subglottic laryngeal stenosis by resection and direct anastomosis. Laryngoscope 84:940–957
2. Pearson FG, Cooper JD, Nelems JM et al (1975) Primary tracheal anastomosis after resection of the cricoid cartilage with preservation of recurrent laryngeal nerves. J Thorac Cardiovasc Surg 70:806–816
3. Monnier P, Savary M, Chapuis G (1993) Partial cricoid resection with primary tracheal anastomosis for subglottic stenosis in infants and children. Laryngoscope 103:1273–1283
4. George M, Ikonomidis C, Jaquet Y et al (2009) Partial cricotracheal resection in children: potential pitfalls and avoidance of complications. Otolaryngol Head Neck Surg 141:225–231
5. Triglia J, Nicollas R, Roman S et al (2000) Cricotracheal resection in children: indications, technique and results. Ann Otolaryngol Chir Cervicofac 117:155–160
6. White DR, Cotton RT, Bean JA et al (2005) Pediatric cricotracheal resection: surgical outcomes and risk factor analysis. Arch Otolaryngol Head Neck Surg 131:896–899

8 Larynx Box

F. Mattioli, G. Mattioli, A. Ghidini, and L. Presutti

8.1 Introduction

Endolaryngeal surgery represents a group of common interventions in otorhinolaryngology, either as a diagnostic technique or as a minimally invasive approach to some laryngeal pathologies. However, the learning curve is steep in view of the limited workspace inside the laryngoscope and the length of the instruments.

A dissection laboratory is a useful educational tool which can be used to rehearse the required specialized surgical skills frequently, particularly in endolaryngeal micro- and laser surgery. However, the availability of fresh human cadavers is limited and may be further restricted by financial or regulatory issues. There is therefore an urgent need for low-cost and easy to handle models or simulators [1].

To this end, the ex vivo animal model is worth considering as fresh animal specimens are widely available at very low cost. Several different animal models have been proposed for endolaryngeal surgery and implemented as models. The histologic comparison of different animal larynges has for some time favored the canine model [2]. Recently, several groups have described and validated the porcine larynx as a suitable candidate [3, 4], which was endorsed by its phonatory properties [5]. The ovine model was also used in recent studies [6] on whole heads, even in training for fibrolaryngoscopy [7]. The choice of a suitable animal model appears to be well investigated and therefore possible.

Hence, a crucial issue to address is the setting of the dissection station. Routinely used for temporal bone dissection, ex vivo laboratories exist in numerous institutions and could host an endolaryngeal dissection station. In endolaryngeal surgery, a lifelike model should include a realistic laryngeal exposure and be comfortable to use, hygienic, and safe with regard to use with a CO_2 laser [8–14].

We designed (Figs. 8.1, 8.2, 8.3, 8.4, 8.5, and 8.6), developed, and validated a dissection station for endolaryngeal surgery (larynx box) suitable for different kinds of larynx (e.g., human, canine, porcine, ovine) and any type of operating technique (CO_2 laser, cold instruments by endoscopic or microscopic techniques). Moreover, it is safe, hygienic, portable, and easy to use.

We constructed a dissection station box from CO_2 laser-resistant material called Makrolon® (Bayer Material Science). It is composed of linear polycarbonate resins and low-viscosity, high-performance thermoplastics, which completely absorb the laser energy. The polycarbonate is bought as flat plates or cylindrical tubes and thereafter cut into the required forms. The cylindrical container of 25 cm diameter is fixed with liquid bicarbonate glue on a footplate of the same material, measuring 40 cm

F. Mattioli (✉) • A. Ghidini • L. Presutti
Head and Neck Department, University Hospital of Modena, Modena, Italy
e-mail: franz318@hotmail.com

G. Mattioli
Private Mechanical Engineer,
Suzzara, Italy

A. Ghidini et al. (eds.), *Atlas of Airway Surgery*, DOI 10.1007/978-3-319-49739-6_8

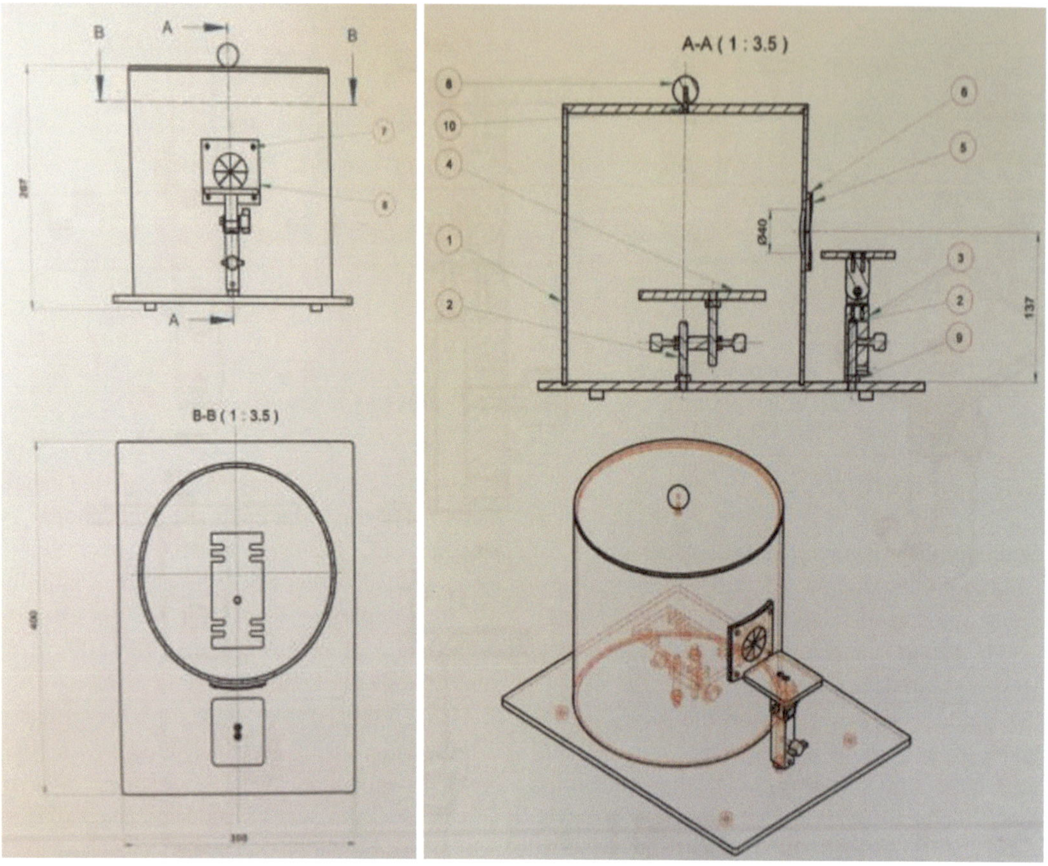

Figs. 8.1 and 8.2 Axial and frontal view of technical draw of the initial prototype of the larynx box

in length and 30 cm width (Figs. 8.7, 8.8, 8.9, and 8.10). Required material thickness is 8 mm for the straight parts and 4 mm for the tube.

The laryngeal support hosted by the dissection station consists of a plate of 13 cm length and 6 cm width, which is articulated for optimal positioning as a function of the laryngeal specimen used (Figs. 8.11 and 8.12).

During dissection, two straps securely fix the larynx (Fig. 8.13). The specimen remains accessible during the whole procedure through the cap on top of the box. An articulated arm mounted on the footplate holds the laryngoscope, which is introduced into the dissection station through a hole covered by a rubber diaphragm. For optimal exposure and an ergonomic setting, the position of the laryngoscope and the laryngeal support may be amended when required. The transparent material allows constant verification of the accurate placement of the specimen, the laryngoscope and instruments during training (Fig. 8.14). Moreover, it guarantees a hygienic work environment since it can easily be cleaned and disinfected after use (even by a machine).

We used our larynx box equipped with a laryngoscope with integrated 0° endoscope (Karl Storz, Tuttlingen, Germany LaryngoFIT HAVAS) (Fig. 8.15) connected to a portable screen with light source (Karl Storz), which was placed in front of the dissector (Figs. 8.16 and 8.17).

The panoramic view of the larynx offered by the endoscope allowed a thorough understanding of the anatomical structures and the teaching steps involved in the different interventions.

Since the ovine model has been described to be suitable for laryngology training [6], we used the larynges of 6-month-old lambs from the local butchery.

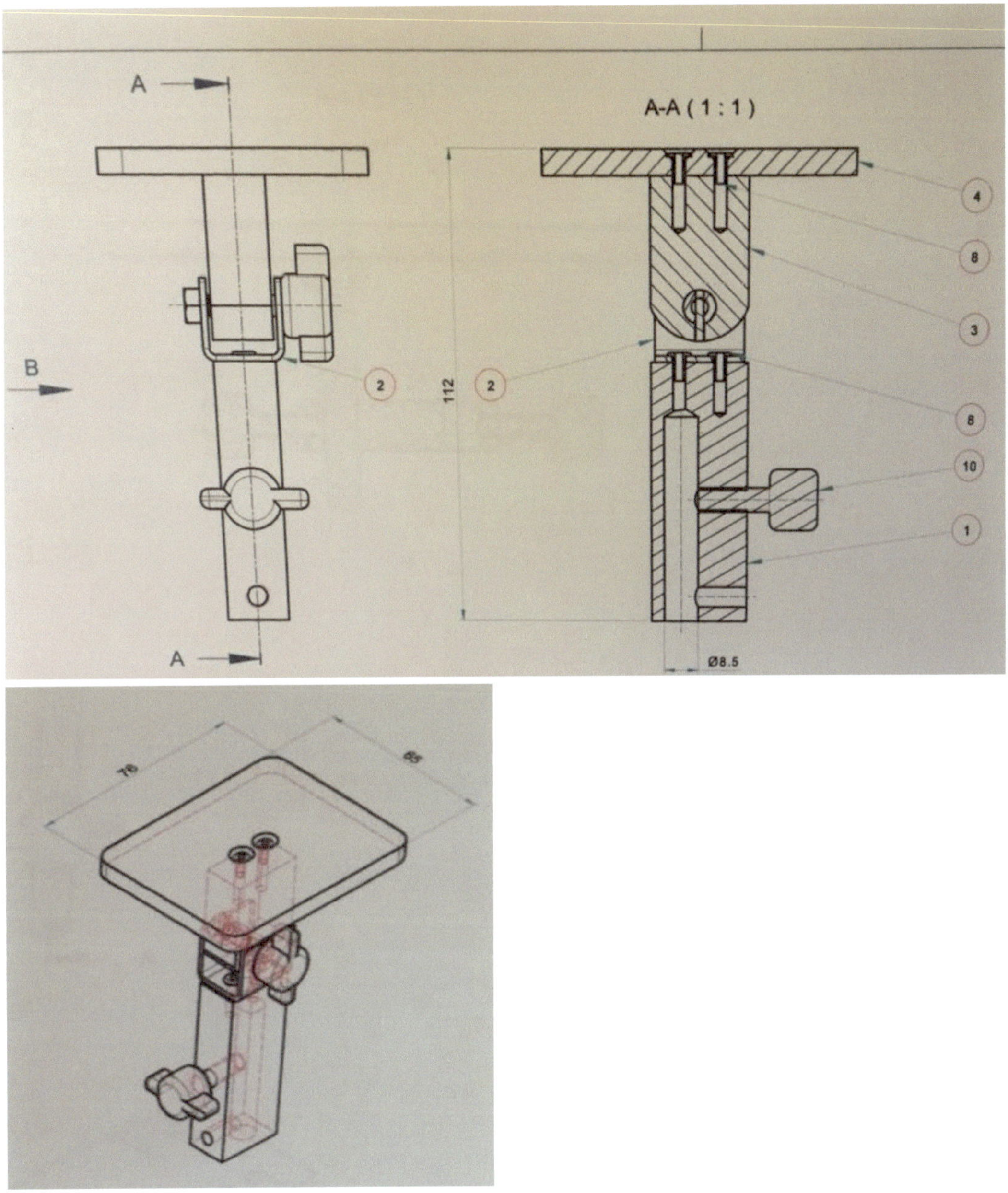

Figs. 8.3 and 8.4 Technical draws of the outer footplate of the larynx box. The footplate has both anteroposterior angle control and height control

The use and safety of the larynx box with use of the CO_2 laser were evaluated in our laboratories. Makrolon is also used in the production of laser protection glasses and is therefore considered to be laser safe. Moreover, polycarbonates are flame retardants and provide additional safety when used with a CO_2 laser. As expected, we did not note any damage or alterations to the dissection station during its use with the CO_2 laser.

After setting up the box as described, we performed the same exercises with cold instruments (cordectomy, arytenoidectomy, posterior cordotomy, and supraglottoplasty) using a Leica F40 microscope and a CO_2 laser.

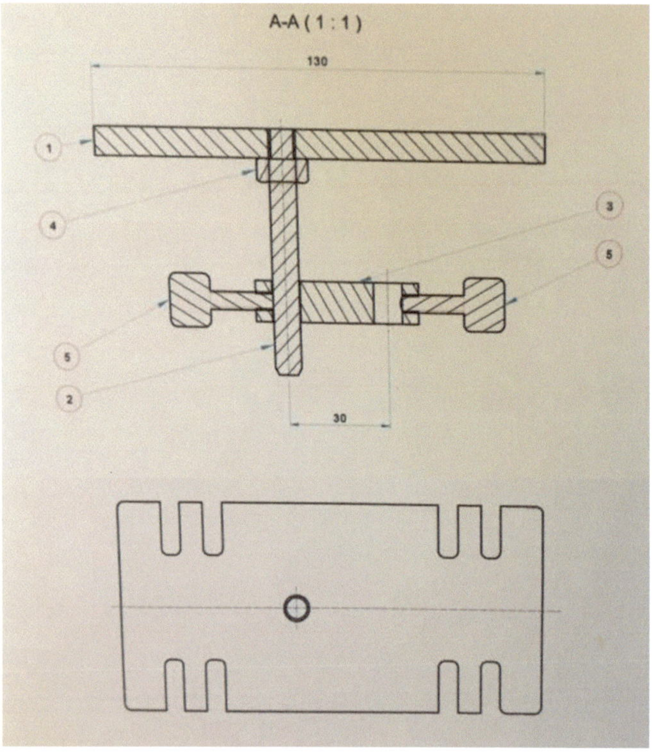

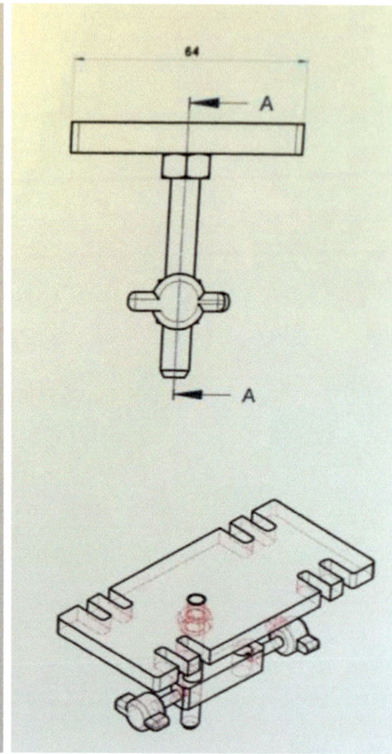

Figs. 8.5 and 8.6 Technical draws of the inner footplate of the larynx box. The inner footplate has both anteroposterior angle control and height control and moreover has several grooves that allow to adjust two straps to securely fix the larynx

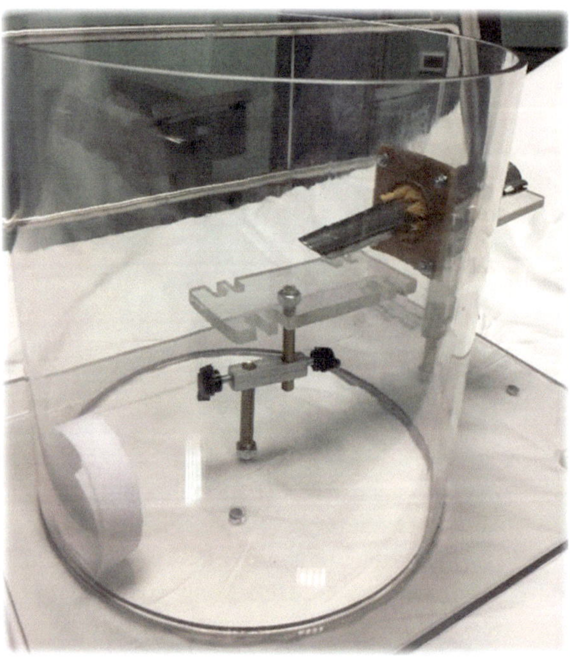

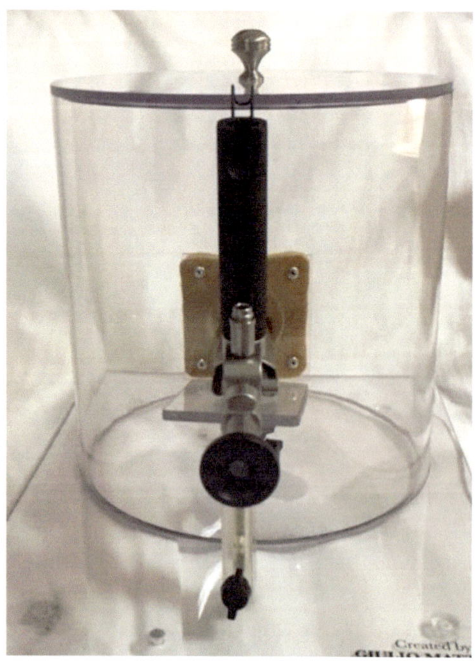

Figs. 8.7 and 8.8 Axial and frontal view of the larynx box

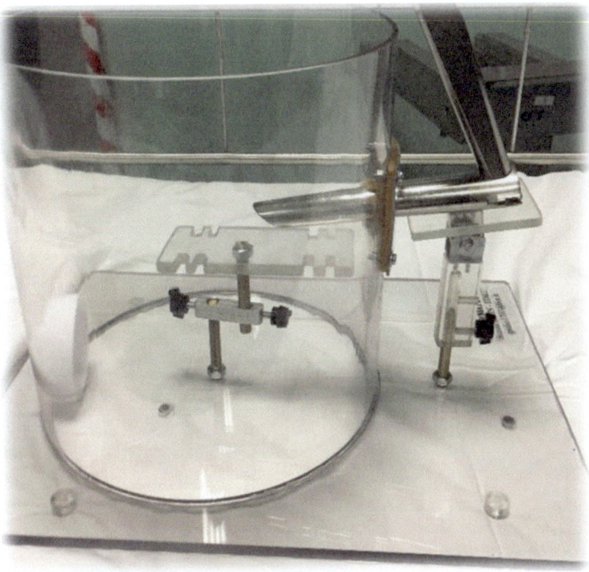
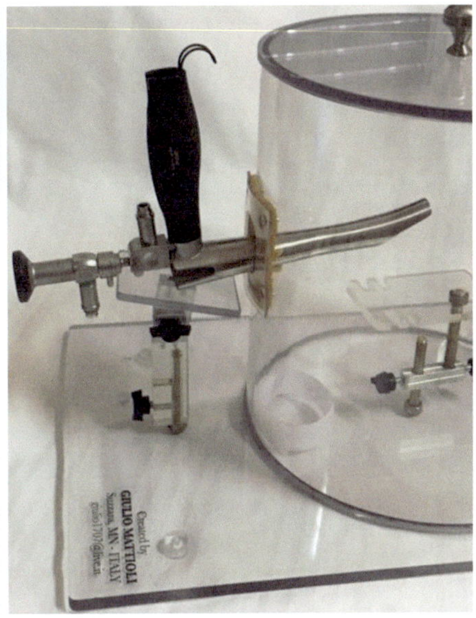

Figs. 8.9 and 8.10 Axial and frontal view of the larynx box equipped with a laryngoscope with integrated 0° endoscope by Storz (LaryngoFIT HAVAS)

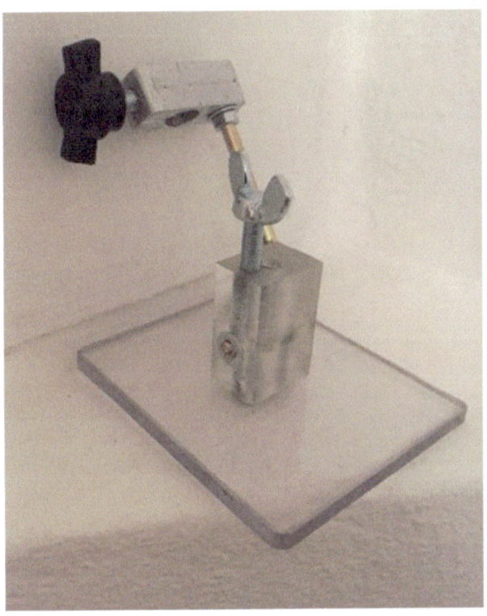
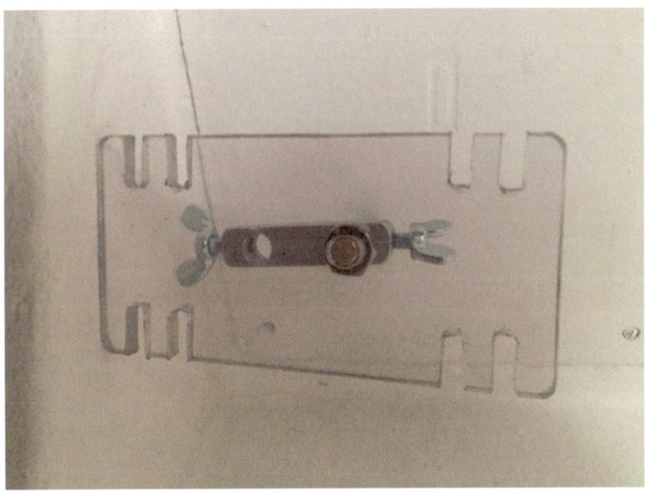

Figs. 8.11 and 8.12 The polycarbonate plates (*inner* and *outer*) which allow a fully stable and secure control of the larynx specimen

The larynx box can be used in the surgery room, perfectly adapted for microscope surgery (Figs. 8.18 and 8.19).

The use of the CO2 laser in endolaryngeal station in use with a microscope. Surgery represents an important aspect of modern surgical approaches and has its own learning curve.12

In our experience, training in the use of a CO2 laser can be easily performed on fresh tissue via the described dissection station. The trainee may improve understanding of tissue reactions to the application of CO2 laser and therefore gain useful experience and not just in the handling of the instruments.

Since the larynx box may be brought to the operating room or a temporal bone dissection laboratory, we may take advantage of already-existing infrastructure for education, which limits additional costs.

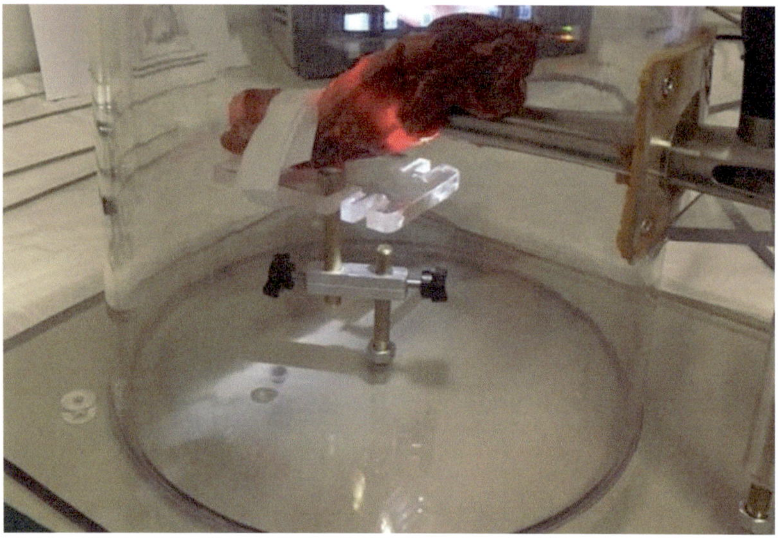

Fig. 8.13 Two straps securely fix the larynx inside the larynx box. The specimen remains accessible during the whole procedure through the cap on top of the box

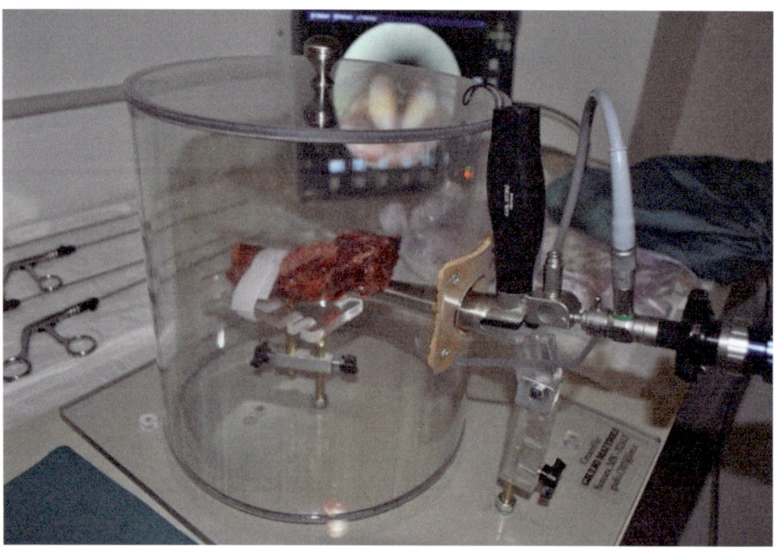

Fig. 8.14 The polycarbonate allows constant verification of the accurate placement of the specimen, the laryngoscope, and instruments during training

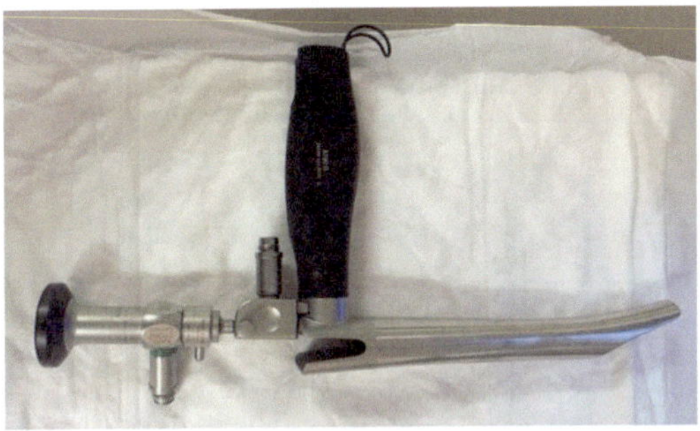

Fig. 8.15 Karl Storz LaryngoFIT HAVAS

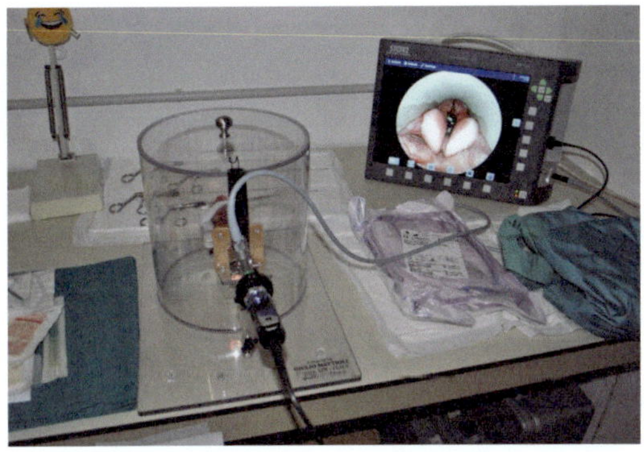

Fig. 8.16 The dissection station with larynx box and connected portable screen

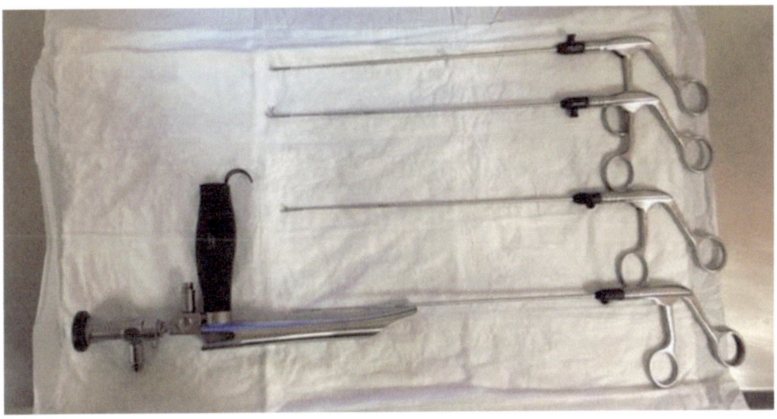

Fig. 8.17 The fully microlaryngo surgery instruments SET by Karl Storz

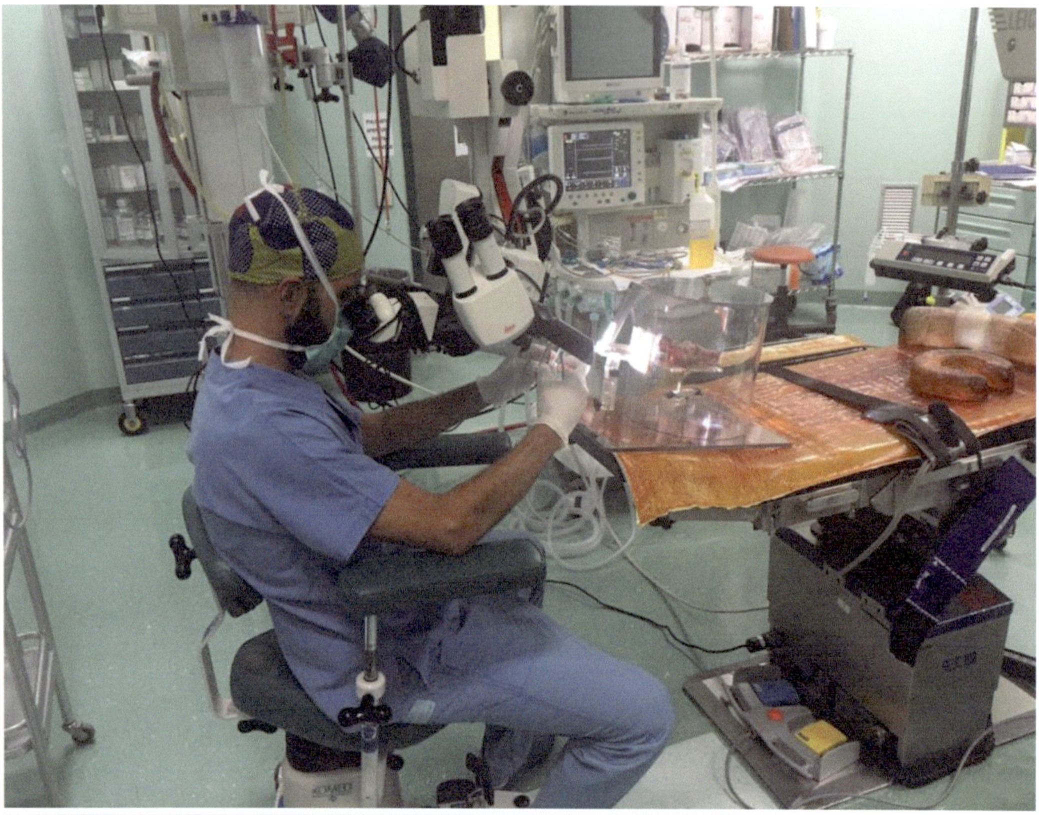

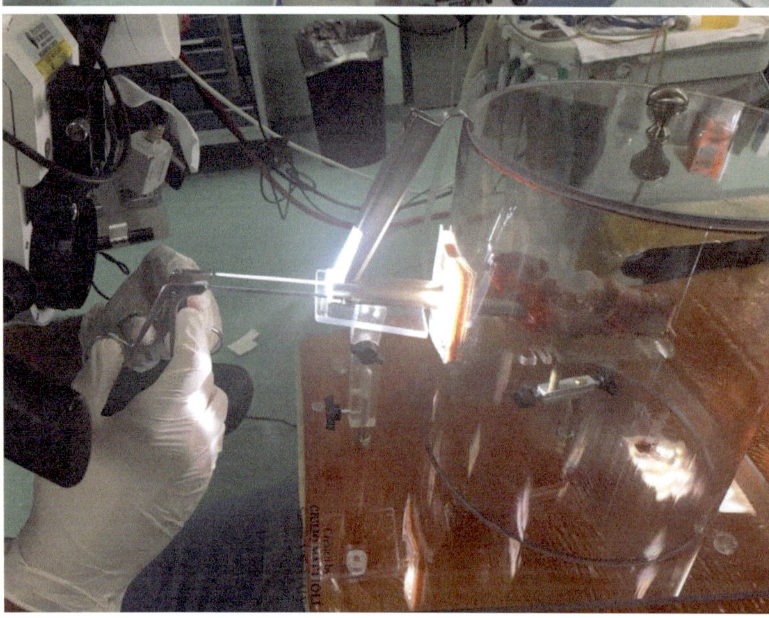

Figs. 8.18 and 8.19 Different angles and overview of the dissecting microscopic setup. A Example of CO2 laser dissection of an ovine larynx

References

1. Gardner AK, Scott DJ, Hebert JC et al (2015) Gearing up for milestones in surgery: will simulation play a role? Surgery 158:1421–1427
2. Garret C, Coleman J, Reinisch L (2000) Comparative histology and vibration of the vocal fold: implications for experimental studies in microlaryngeal surgery. Laryngoscope 110:814–824
3. Nasser KM, Wahba HA, Kamal E, El-Makhzangy AM, Bahaa N (2012) Animal model for training and improvement of the surgical skills in endolaryngeal microsurgery. J Voice 26:351–357
4. Dedmon MM, Paddle PM, Phillips J, Kobayashi L, Franco RA, Song PC (2015) Development and validation of a high-fidelity porcine laryngeal surgical simulator. Otolaryngol Head Neck Surg 153:420–426
5. Jiang JJ, Raviv JR, Hanson DG (2001) Comparison of the phonation related structures among pig, dog, white-tailed deer, and human larynges. Ann Otol Rhinol Laryngol 110:1120–1125
6. Ianacone DC, Gnadt BJ, Isaacson G (2016) Ex vivo ovine model for head and neck surgical simulation. Am J Otolaryngol 37:272–278
7. Isaacson G, Ianacone DC, Wolfson MR (2015) Ex vivo ovine model for pediatric flexible endoscopy training. Int J Pediatr Otorhinolaryngol 79: 2196–2199
8. Paczona R (1997) A cadaver larynx holder for teaching laryngomicrosurgery. J Laryngol Otol 111:56–57
9. Mohamed AS, McCulloch TM (2004) A larynx holder: a device for training in microlaryngeal surgery. Laryngoscope 114:1128–1129
10. Verma SP, Dailey SH, McMurray JS, Jiang JJ, McCulloch TM (2010) Implementation of a program for surgical education in laryngology. Laryngoscope 120:2241–2246
11. Nixon IJ, Palmer FL, Ganly I, Patel SG (2012) An integrated simulator for endolaryngeal surgery. Laryngoscope 122:140–143
12. Hartl DM, Brasnu DF (2015) Contemporary surgical management of early glottic cancer. Otolaryngol Clin North Am 48:611–625
13. Stasche N, Quirrenbach T, Barmann M, Krebs M, Harrass M, Friedrich K (2005) IMOLA: a new larynx model for surgical training.Education in transoral laser microsurgery of the upper airways. HNO 53:869–872 874-865
14. Awad Z, Patel B, Hayden L, Sandhu GS, Tolley NS (2015) Simulationin laryngology training; what should we invest in? Our experiencewith 64 porcine larynges and a literature review. Clin Otolaryngol 40:269–273

Endoscopic Procedures

9

M.P. Alberici, M. Menichetti,
E. Aggazzotti Cavazza, S. Bottero, A. Ghidini,
and L. Presutti

9.1 Introduction

Endoscopic procedures include vocal cordotomy, arytenoidectomy, endoscopic mucosal advancement flap, and endoscopic posterior cricoid split with rib grafting [1]. The use of lasers in endoscopic procedures is relatively recent [2]. In this chapter, these techniques will be illustrated step by step, made on sheep's larynx, using CO2 laser or cold instruments.

9.1.1 Indication

The main indication to this type of surgery is bilateral vocal fold immobility (BVFI) with and without laryngeal stenosis both in pediatric and adult populations. BVFI can be divided into bilateral vocal fold paralysis (BVFP) and cricoarytenoid joint fixation (CAJF), which can be accompanied with posterior glottic stenosis (PGS) and/or subglottic stenosis (SGS). Many children with BVFI resulting in upper airway obstruction will require a tracheostomy [1].

M.P. Alberici (✉) • M. Menichetti
E. Aggazzotti Cavazza • A. Ghidini
L. Presutti
Head and Neck Department,
University Hospital of Modena, Modena, Italy
e-mail: maria.paola.alberici@alice.it

S. Bottero
Airway Surgery Unit, Laryngotracheal Team Director,
Bambino Gesù Children's Hospital, Rome, Italy

Others possible procedures that can be used in BVFI are open procedures that include scar excision, mucosal grafts/flaps with and without stenting, and laryngotracheal reconstruction.

The decision to perform an endoscopic procedure vs an open surgery is based on the ability to obtain good endoscopic exposure, and also endoscopic approaches are preferred when possible due to less morbidity resulting in a faster recovery [1].

9.1.2 Contraindication

These procedures should be avoided in case of poor endoscopic exposure of the larynx (e.g., retrognathia, micrognathia, glossoptosis, macroglossia) or retroflexion of the epiglottis or severe transglottic stenosis or Grade 4 SGS.

9.1.3 Instrumentation and Equipment

If possible it is better to work in pairs.

Before starting your laboratory session, you should have these materials on hand:

- Dissection tray or a diaper
- Endoscopic tools: one Telepack X LED (Storz®) (Fig. 9.1a); one operating laryngoscope (HAVAS Operating Laryngoscope Storz® with light carrier) (Fig. 9.1b); one

A. Ghidini et al. (eds.), *Atlas of Airway Surgery*, DOI 10.1007/978-3-319-49739-6_9

straightforward telescope 0° (Hopkins II® – Storz®) (Fig. 9.1b); three laryngeal forceps (LaryngoFIT HAVAS® – Storz®) (Fig.9.1c), one with bite spoon (Fig. 9.2c), one fluted straight (Fig. 9.2d), and one triangular fluted straight (Fig. 9.2b); one laryngeal scissor (LaryngoFIT HAVAS® – Storz®) (Fig. 9.2a); one laser CO_2

- Medical gauzes
- Paper towel

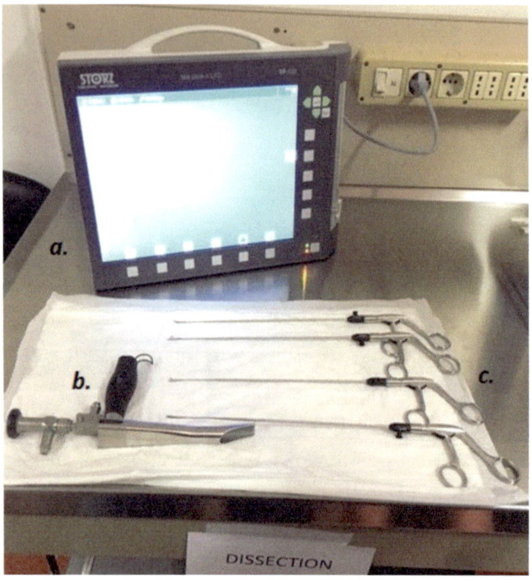

Fig. 9.1 Endoscopic tools: (**a**) Telepack X LED (Storz®). (**b**) operating laryngoscope (HAVAS Operating Laryngoscope Storz® with light carrier) and one straightforward telescope 0° (Hopkins II® – Storz®). (**c**) three laryngeal forceps (LaryngoFIT HAVAS® – Storz®)

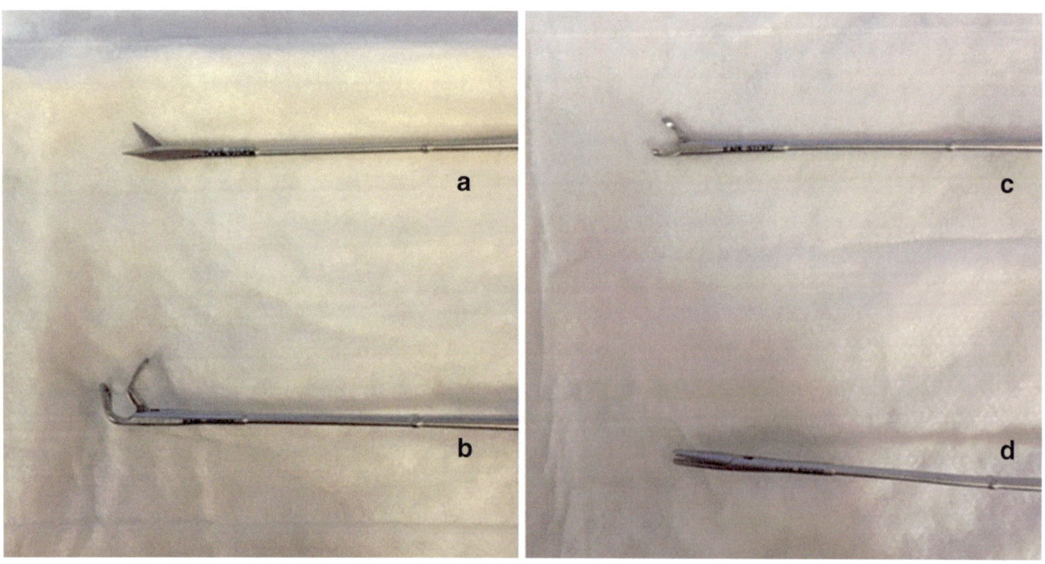

Fig. 9.2 Endoscopic tools: (**a**) laryngeal scissor (LaryngoFIT HAVAS® – Storz®). (**b**) triangular fluted straight. (**c**) one with bite spoon. (**d**) one fluted straight

9.2 Arytenoidectomy

Arytenoidectomy is a permanent and irreversible surgical procedure where the laryngeal inlet is widened in its transverse axis. The aim is to enlarge the glottic airway size to improve symptoms, with minimal adverse effect on voice and swallowing [3].

Arytenoidectomy is usually performed in cases of bilateral vocal fold immobility caused by either paralysis of the vocal cords or their fixation [4, 5]. It may be divided into a conservative procedure (transverse cordotomy and medial arytenoidectomy) and a radical procedure (total arytenoidectomy) [6]. *Ossoff* et al. described the total (complete) arytenoidectomy procedure in 1983 [4]. *Dennis* and *Kashima* first described the procedure of transverse cordotomy or posterior cordectomy in 1989 [7]. Medial arytenoidectomy (partial arytenoidectomy) was described in 1993 by Crumley [8].

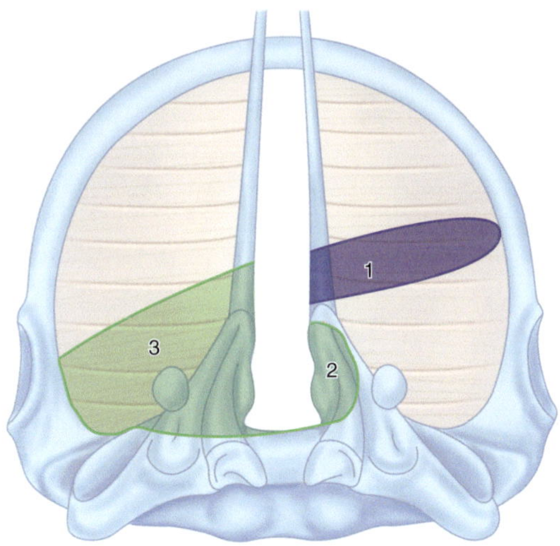

Fig. 9.3 Different degrees of arytenoid removal (medial, total) compared with transverse cordotomy: Area n.1: transverse cordotomy; Area n.2: laser ablation of the medial arytenoid for medial arytenoidectomy; Area n.3: laser ablation of total arytenoidectomy

Arytenoidectomy can be performed endoscopically by conventional cold steel microsurgery or with the use of laser; currently, the latter is the more popular approach [5, 9, 10]. Endoscopic partial arytenoidectomy and posterior/transverse cordotomy have become more popular recently, because it was claimed that total arytenoidectomy led to aspiration problems postoperatively and disturbed voice significantly [11].

Arytenoidectomy can also be done by an external or open method if laser is not available, if previous endoscopic or microsurgical procedures have failed, or in cases for which access to the area is limited by anatomical distortions (Fig. 9.3).

Different degrees of arytenoid removal (medial, total) compared with transverse cordotomy:

Area n.1: transverse cordotomy
Area n.2: laser ablation of the medial arytenoid for medial arytenoidectomy
Area n.3: laser ablation of total arytenoidectomy

9.2.1 Arytenoidectomy with Laser [12]

Step 1

- Exposition of glottic area, especially its posterior portion (Fig. 9.4).
- An incision along the arytenoid mucosa is marked with CO_2 laser spots. CO_2 laser is used at 5-W power, with the smallest spot size available and continuous mode to make a mucosal incision down until arytenoid cartilage is reached. (Figs. 9.5, 9.6 and 9.7)

Step 2

- Submucosal dissection of the cartilage is performed using CO2 laser.
- Arytenoid cartilage is dissected off the surrounding tissues using also microscissor. The junction of arytenoid with cricoid is identified, and that is the posterior wall of the joint capsule. The joint is opened. The arytenoid is removed from the cricoid cartilage by the use of laser CO2 (Figs. 9.8, 9.9, 9.10 and 9.11)

Step 3

In order to avoid stenosis and granuloma formation, the area which corresponds to arytenoidectomy is recovered by repositioning of mucosal flap with Vicryl 4.0 suture and fibrin adhesive.

The medially based advancement flap is sutured posterolaterally endoscopically between the anterior edge of the mucosal flap and the surgical bed (H) around the previous place of the muscular process of arytenoid (Figs. 9.12 and 9.13).

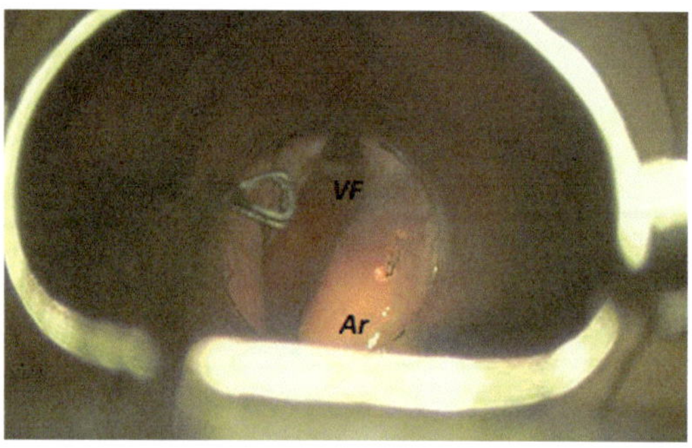

Fig. 9.4 *Ar* arytenoid, *VF* vocal fold

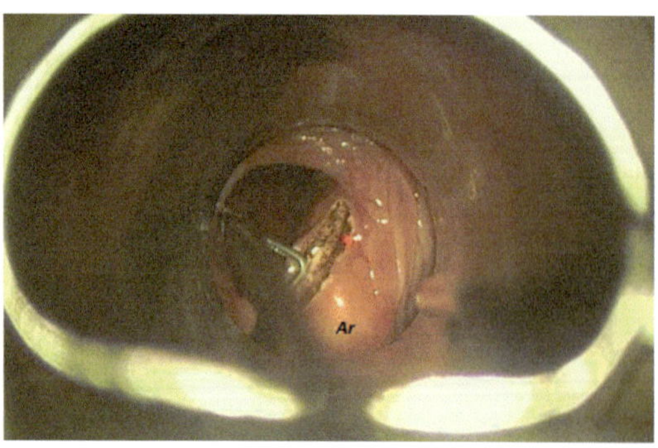

Fig. 9.5 *Ar* arytenoid

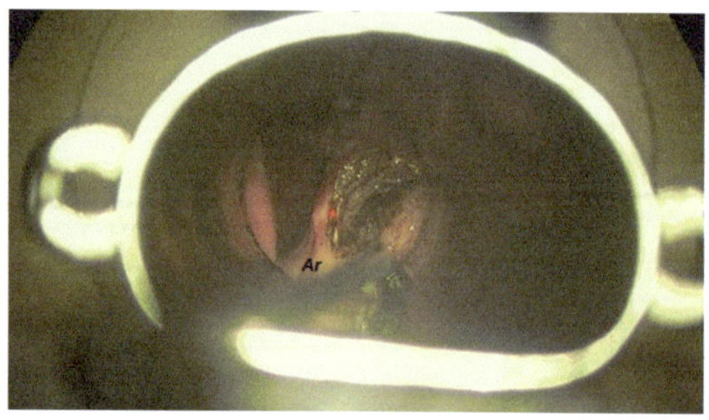

Fig. 9.6 *Ar* arytenoid

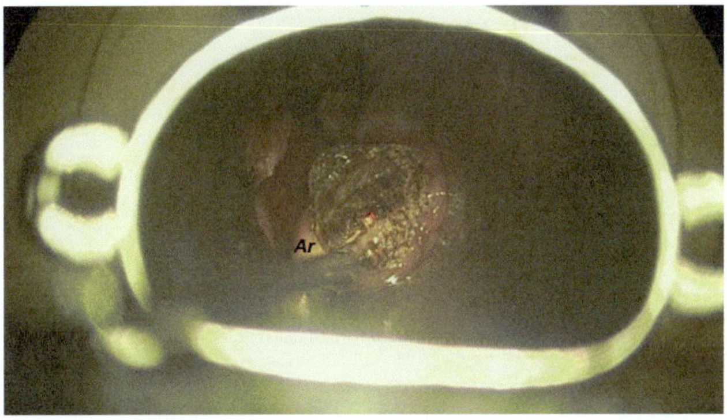

Fig. 9.7 *Ar* arytenoid

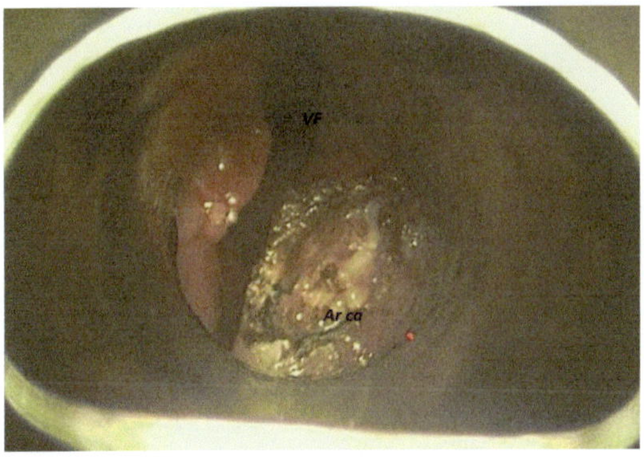

Fig. 9.8 Ar ca arytenoid cartilage

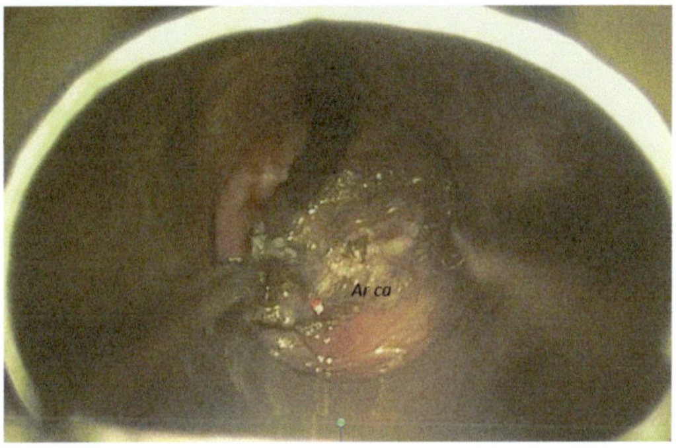

Fig. 9.10 *Ar ca* arytenoid cartilage

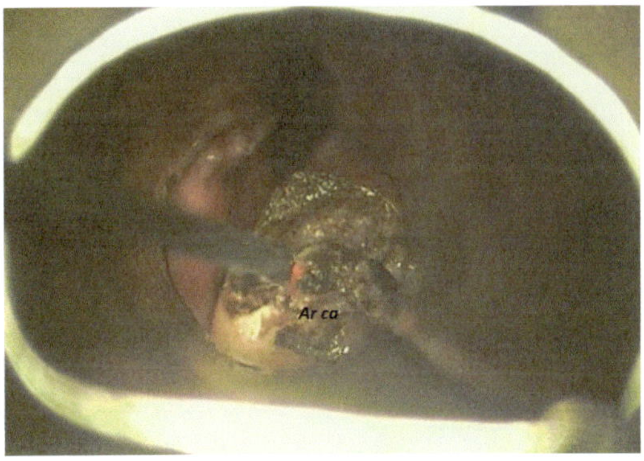

Fig. 9.9 Ar ca arytenoid cartilage

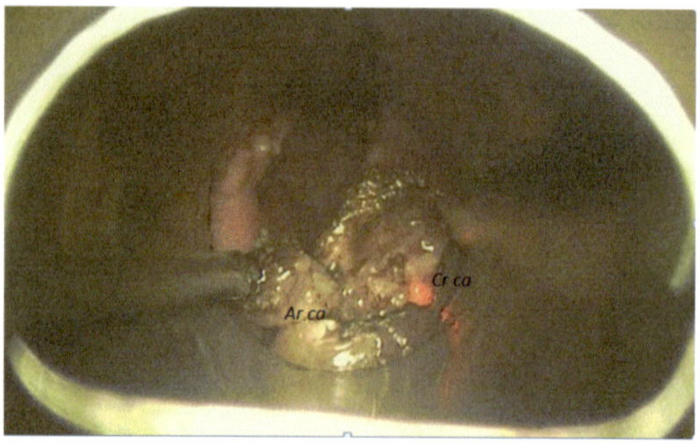

Fig. 9.11 *Ar ca* arytenoid cartilage, *Cr ca* cricoid cartilage

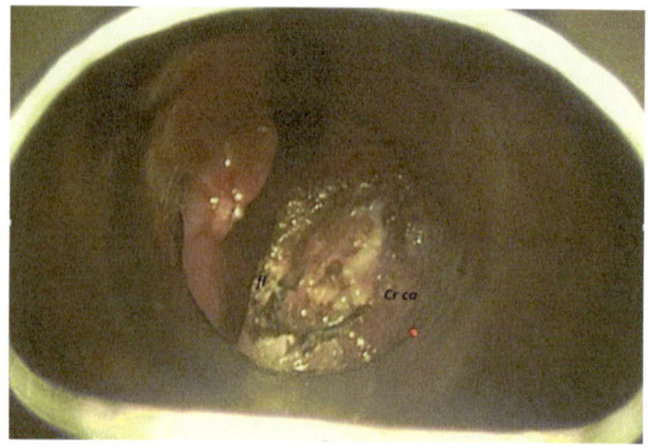

Fig. 9.12 fl mucosal flap, Cr ca cricoid cartilage

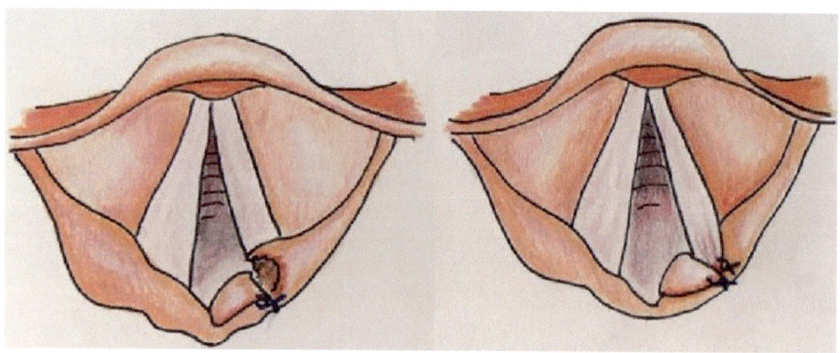

Fig. 9.13 The area which corresponds to arytenoidectomy is recovered by repositioning of mucosal flap with Vicryl 4.0 suture and fibrin adhesive

9.2.1.1 Arytenoidectomy with Cold Instruments

Step 1

- Exposition of glottic area, especially its posterior portion (Fig. 9.14).
- Start to cut with microscissors the arytenoid mucosa in the lateral face (Fig. 9.15).
- Start the submucosal dissection of the cartilage with microscissors (Figs. 9.16 and 9.17).

Step 2

- Arytenoid cartilage is dissected off the surrounding tissues. The muscular process of arytenoid is sharply dissected off its muscular attachments (Figs. 9.18 and 9.19).
- The junction of arytenoid with cricoid is identified, and that is the posterior wall of the joint capsule. The joint is opened. The arytenoid is removed from the cricoid cartilage by cutting other connective tissue components of the joint (Fig. 9.20).

Step 3

In order to avoid stenosis and granuloma formation, the area which corresponds to arytenoidectomy is recovered by repositioning of mucosal flap with Vicryl 4.0 suture and fibrin adhesive. The medially based advancement flap is sutured posterolaterally endoscopically between the anterior edge of the mucosal flap and the surgical bed around the previous place of the muscular process of arytenoid (Figs. 9.21 and 9.22).

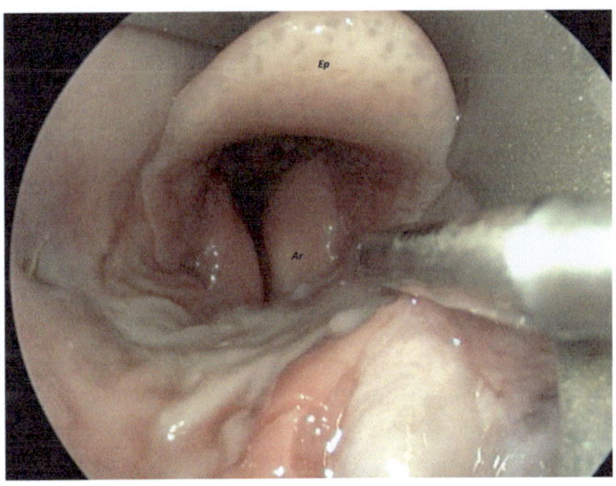

Fig. 9.14 *Ep* epiglottis, *Ar ca* arytenoid cartilage, *Ar mu* arytenoid mucosa

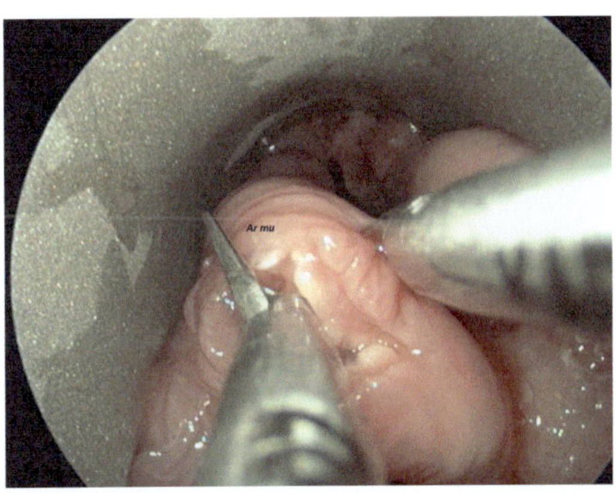

Fig. 9.15 *Ar mu* arytenoid mucosa

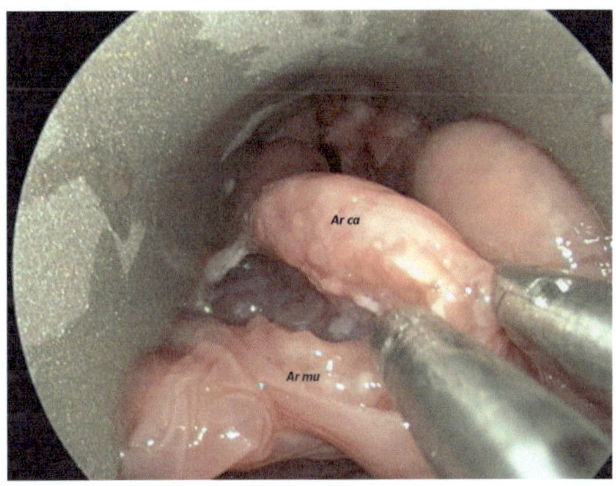

Fig. 9.16 *Ar ca* arytenoid cartilage, *Ar mu* arytenoid mucosa

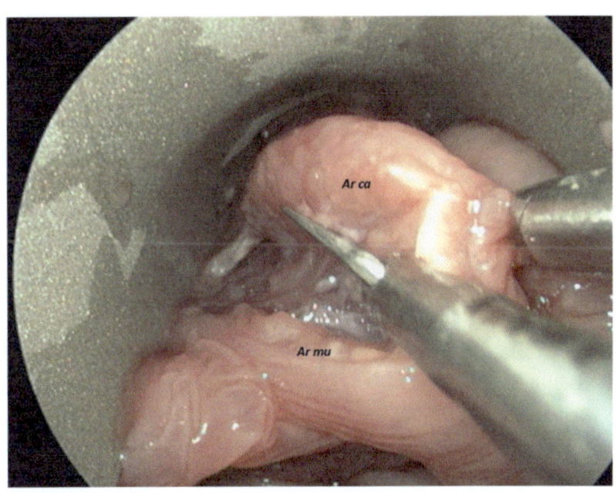

Fig. 9.17 *Ar ca* arytenoid cartilage, *Ar mu* arytenoid mucosa

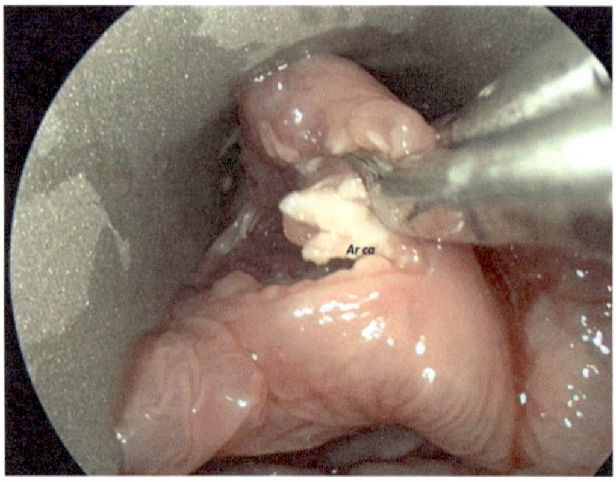

Fig. 9.18 *Ar ca* arytenoid

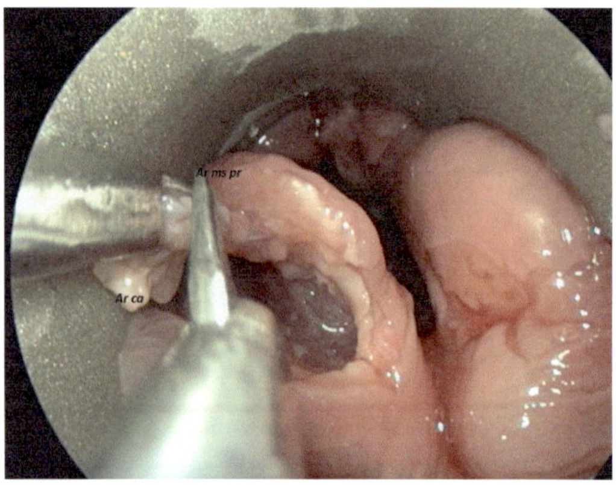

Fig. 9.19 *Ar ca* arytenoid, *Ar ms pr* muscular process of arytenoid

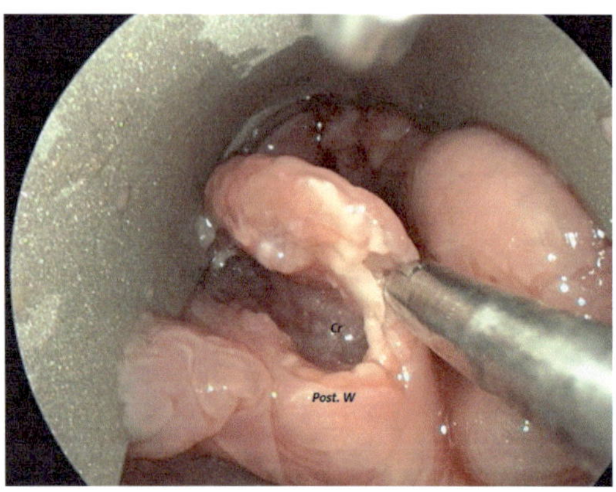

Fig. 9.20 *Cr* cricoid, *Post W* posterior wall of the joint capsule

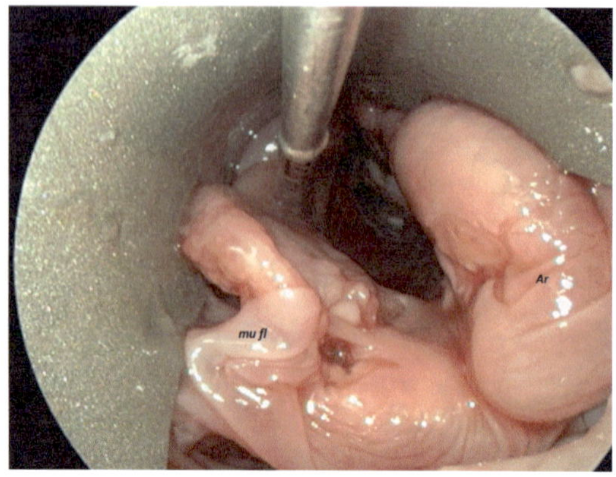

Fig. 9.21 *mu fl* mucosal flap, *Ar* arytenoid

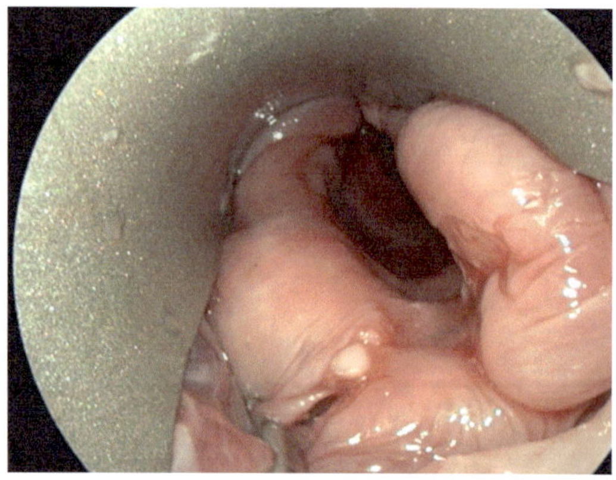

Fig. 9.22 The medially based advancement flap is sutured posterolaterally endoscopically between the anterior edge of the mucosal flap and the surgical bed around the previous place of the muscular process of arytenoid

9.3 Posterior Cricoid Split

Airway enlargement by way of cricoid expansion with cartilage augmentation is one approach to correct laryngeal airway obstruction at the glottic and subglottic levels [13]. Expansion of the posterior aspect of the cricoid with costal cartilage grafting as a component of laryngotracheal reconstruction has been extensively described in the literature, in particular in children [14].

In 1994, *Gray* et al. first described the use of isolated posterior cricoid split and costal cartilage graft placement for bilateral vocal fold paralysis (BVFP) [15].

Step 1
Create the graft (Fig. 9.23)

Step 2

- Lindholm or Parsons laryngoscope is used with the laryngeal spreader placed in an inverted fashion and suspended from the laryngoscope.
- Setup operating microscope with CO2 laser adaptor and micromanipulator – 5 W and pulse mode The CO2 laser at a 4- to 8-watt super-pulse mode is used to make a vertical midline incision in the posterior cricoid plate
- Posterior and inferior pressure on the upper aspect of the posterior cricoid is important to obtain an adequate angle for the laser on the posterior cricoid plate and avoid injury to the interarytenoid musculature [15]. It is important to cut the entire length of the cricoids and to not cut through the posterior perichondrium and to do not undermine perichondrium once through the cricoids.

Step 3
The graft size is based on the measurement of the length of the cricoid and width of the expanded posterior split. After creating a lateral trough approximately 1.5 mm deep in the graft, the inner 1 mm edge of each side of the trough is removed, giving the final keyhole shape of the graft similar. A monofilament suture is temporarily placed.

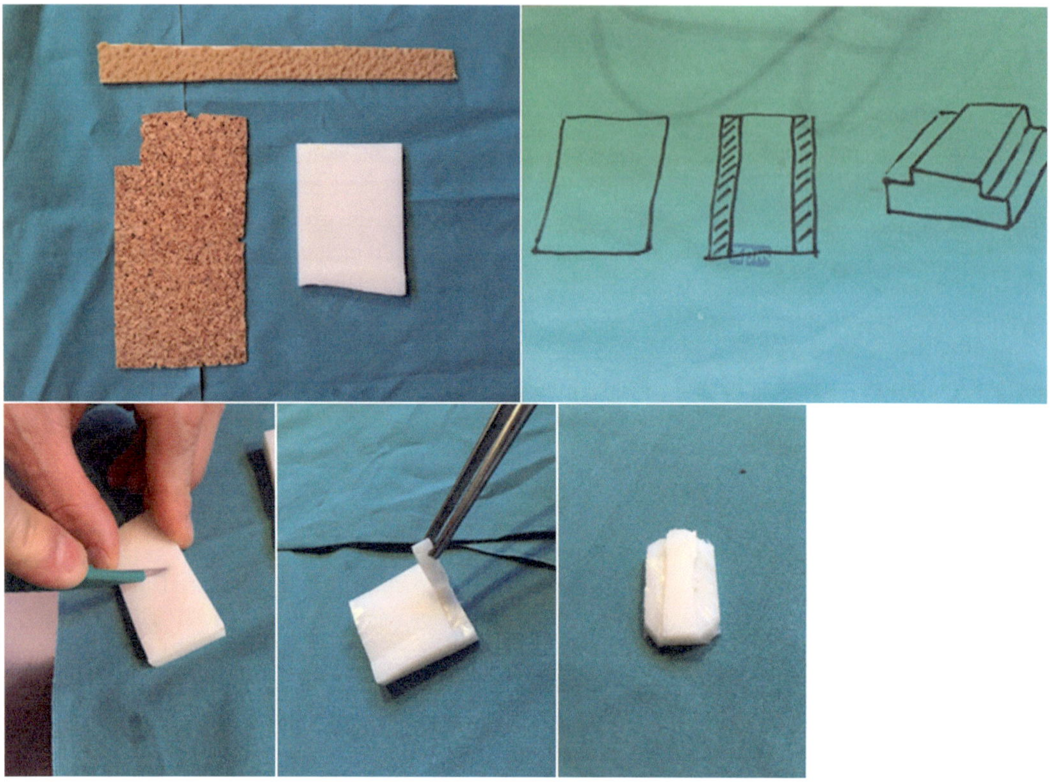

Fig. 9.23 How to create a graft (see also Chap. 4); measure of the graft 10 × 5 × 4 mm

9.4 Posterior Cordotomy with Laser

Posterior cordotomy with the use of laser is a minimal invasive procedure done for the bilateral vocal fold paralysis in midline position [16].

Laser cordectomy was first described in 1989 by Kashima [7]. In 1999, Friedman et al. described the application of the cordotomy in children from 14 months to 13 years old [17]. The technique was effective and associated with good functional results [16] (Fig. 9.24).

Steps (Figs. 9.25, 9.26, 9.27 and 9.28)

- Exposition of glottic area, especially its posterior portion. In vivo it can be used as a palpator in order to discard fixation of arytenoid cartilage and posterior glottis stenosis.
- Cordotomy is performed using a CO2 laser, with 0.2 mm spot size and a power setting of 3–5 watts, by sectioning the vocal cord, 1–2 mm anterior to the vocal process, before the vocal process of arytenoid, transectioning mucosa, vocal ligament, and fibers of thyroarytenoid muscle in lateral way.

The cordotomy both opens the air way posteriorly and provides access to the arytenoid cartilage. Postoperatively, patient is maintained on antibiotics and antireflux medications until mucosal healing is complete.

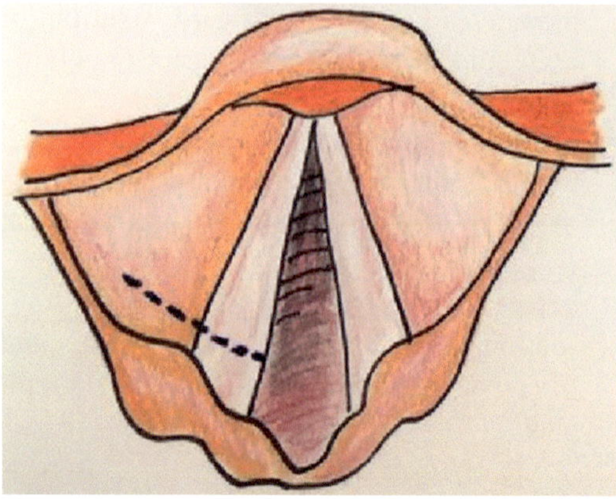

Fig. 9.24 Posterior laser cordotomy

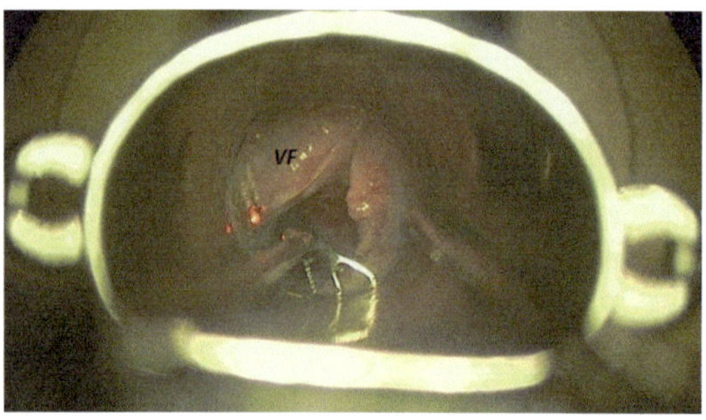

Fig. 9.25 Exposition of glottic area, especially its posterior portion

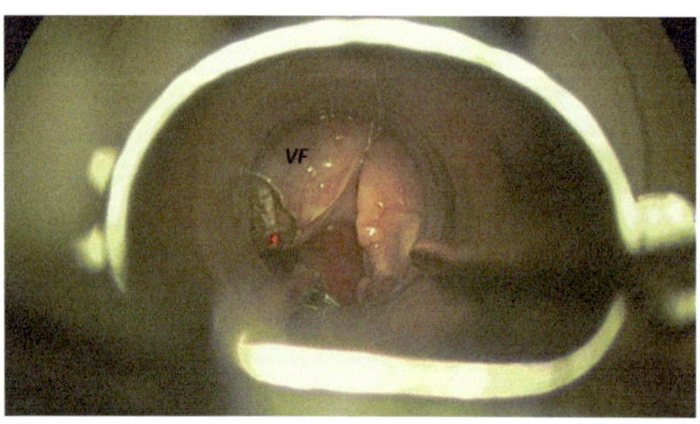

Fig. 9.26 *VF* Vocal fold

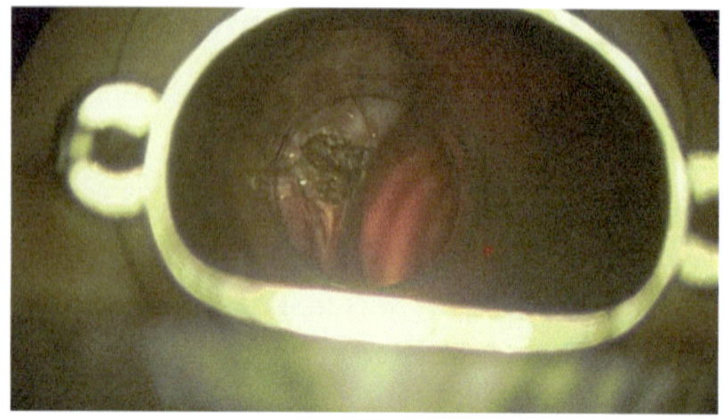

Fig. 9.27 Cordotomy is performed using a CO_2 laser by sectioning the vocal cord, 1–2 mm anterior to the vocal process

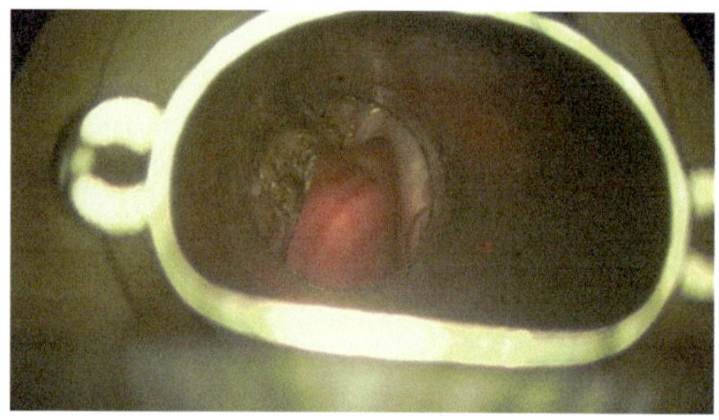

Fig. 9.28 Cordotomy is performed before the vocal process of arytenoid, transectioning mucosa, vocal ligament, and fibers of thyroarytenoid muscle in lateral way

9.5 Supraglottoplasty

Endoscopic supraglottoplasty is the current mainstay and first-line operation for infants with severe laryngomalacia [18].

This procedure was first described by Zalzal et al. in 1987 using cold instruments [19]. Subsequently, the carbon dioxide laser became popular, and since then, the microdebrider has been introduced [20, 21]. Recent studies suggest that there is no difference in outcome between the two endoscopic instrumentation (laser vs cold steel) techniques [22, 23] (Fig. 9.29).

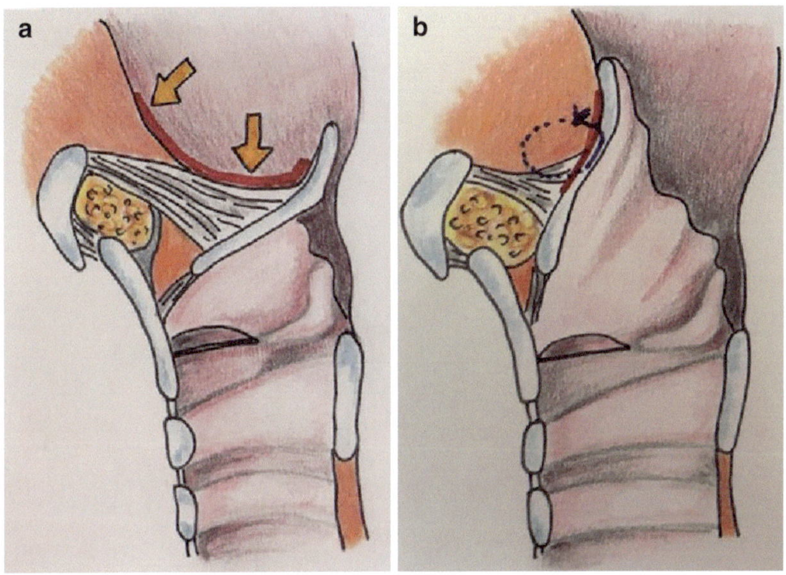

Fig. 9.29 Schematic supraglottoplasty used for type III laryngomalacia: (**a**) An incision using CO_2 laser is created on the base of tongue and lingual aspect of the epiglottis (*yellow arrows*). (**b**) An epiglottopexy is performed, using 4.0 Vicryl sutures to stitch the epiglottis to the tongue base with an endoscopic needle holder

9.5.1 Supraglottoplasty with Laser

Steps

- Divide the aryepiglottic fold with microlaryngeal scissors and resect with laser (Figs. 9.30 and 9.31).
- Cut with laser from anteriorly to the lateral edge of the epiglottis and posteriorly to the arytenoid cartilage (Fig. 9.32).
- Remove the redundant supra-arytenoid mucosa (Fig. 9.33).
- Perform the epiglottopexy, using 4.0 Vicryl sutures to stitch the epiglottis to the tongue base with an endoscopic needle holder.

The interarytenoid space must absolutely not be violated to prevent the development of interarytenoid scarring and posterior glottic fixation.

Take-Home Message

Sheep neck has great similarities with humans in size of the organs, and it is a cheap and practical model which can be used to learn in particular endoscopic procedures, by using an adequate support like larynx box (see Chap. 8). You can perform the endoscopic technique by using laser or with cold instrument.

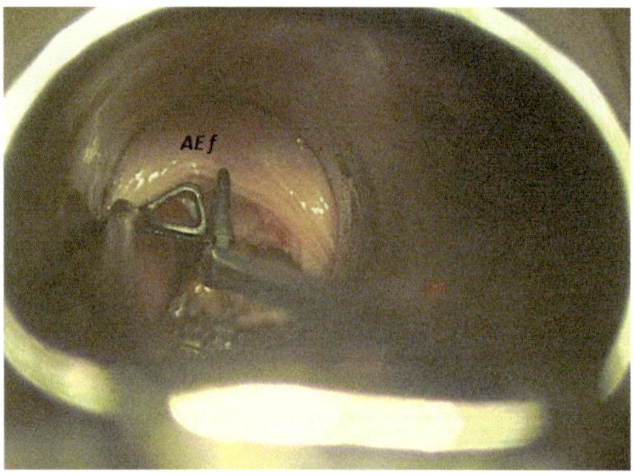

Fig. 9.30 *AEf* aryepiglottic fold

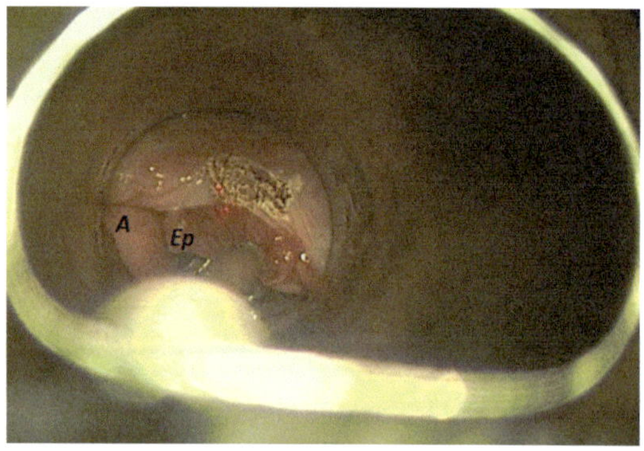

Fig. 9.32 *A* arytenoid, *Ep* epiglottis

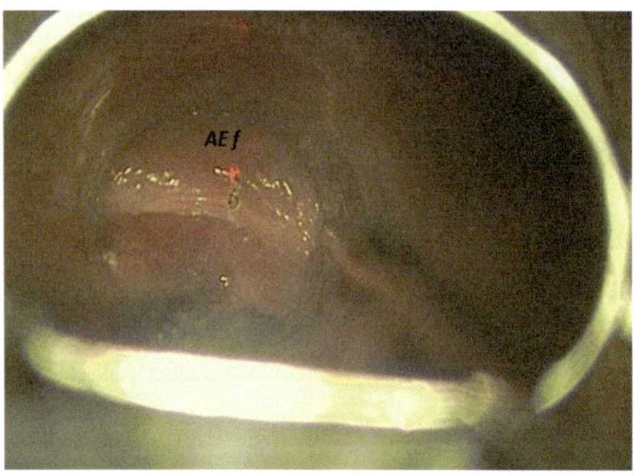

Fig. 9.31 *AEf* aryepiglottic fold

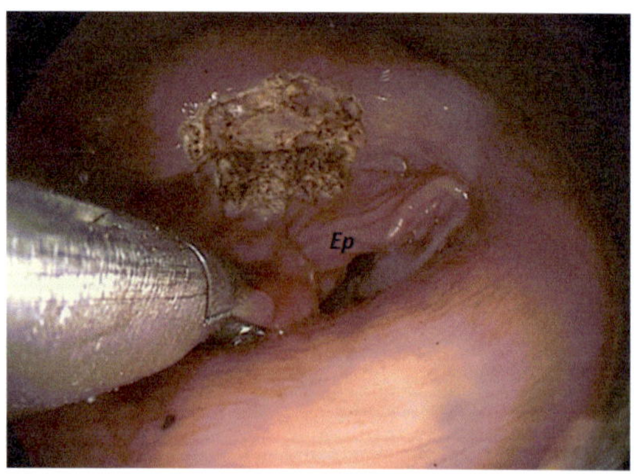

Fig. 9.33 *Ep* epiglottis

References

1. Modi VK (2012) Endoscopic posterior cricoid split with rib grafting. Adv Otorhinolaryngol 73:116–122. doi:10.1159/000334463 Epub 2012 Mar 29. Review
2. Yan Y, Olszewski AE, Hoffman MR, Zhuang P, Ford CN, Dailey SH, Jiang JJ (2010) Use of lasers in laryngeal surgery. J Voice 24(1):102–109
3. Young VN, Rosen CA (2011) Arytenoid and posterior vocal fold surgery for bilateral vocal fold immobility. Curr Opin Otolaryngol Head Neck Surg 19(6):422–427
4. Ossoff RH, Sisson GA, Duncavage JA, Moselle HI, Andrews PE, McMillan WG (1984) Endoscopic laser arytenoidectomy for the treatment of bilateral vocal cord paralysis. Laryngoscope 94(10):1293–1297
5. Aubry K, Leboulanger N, Harris R, Genty E, Denoyelle F, Garabedian EN (2010) Laser arytenoidectomy in the management of bilateral vocal cord paralysis in children. Int J Pediatr Otorhinolaryngol 74(5):451–455
6. Bosley B, Rosen CA, Simpson CB, McMullin BT, Gartner-Schmidt JL (2005) Medial arytenoidectomy versus transverse cordotomy as a treatment for bilateral vocal fold paralysis. Ann Otol Rhinol Laryngol 114(12):922–926
7. Dennis DP, Kashima H (1989) Carbon dioxide laser posterior cordectomy for treatment of bilateral vocal cord paralysis. Ann Otol Rhinol Laryngol 98(12 Pt 1):930–934
8. Crumley RL (1993) Endoscopic laser medial arytenoidectomy for airway management in bilateral laryngeal paralysis. Ann Otol Rhinol Laryngol 102(2):81–84
9. Al-Fattah HA, Hamza A, Gaafar A, Tantawy A (2006) Partial laser arytenoidectomy in the management of bilateral vocal fold immobility: a modification based on functional anatomical study of the cricoarytenoid joint. Otolaryngol Head Neck Surg 134(2):294–301
10. Sato K, Umeno H, Nakashima T (2001) Laser arytenoidectomy for bilateral median vocal fold fixation. Laryngoscope 111:168–171
11. Dursun G, Gokcan K (2006) Aerodynamic, acoustic and functional results of posterior transverse laser cordotomy for bilateral abductor vocal fold paralysis. J Laryngol Otol 120:282–288
12. Yilmaz T (2012) Endoscopic total arytenoidectomy for bilateral abductor vocal fold paralysis: a new flap technique and personal experience with 50 cases. Laryngoscope 122(10):2219–2226
13. Inglis AF Jr, Perkins JA, Manning SC, Mouzakes J (2003) Endoscopic posterior cricoid split and rib grafting in 10 children. Laryngoscope 113(11):2004–2009
14. Gerber ME, Modi VK, Ward RF, Gower VM, Thomsen J (2013) Endoscopic posterior cricoid split and costal cartilage graft placement in children. Otolaryngol Head Neck Surg 148(3):494–502
15. Gray SD, Kelly SM, Dove H (1994) Arytenoid separation for impaired pediatric vocal fold mobility. Ann Otol Rhinol Laryngol 103:510–515
16. Lagier A, Nicollas R, Sanjuan M, Benoit L, Triglia JM (2009) Laser cordotomy for the treatment of bilateral vocal cord paralysis in infants. Int J Pediatr Otorhinolaryngol 73(1):9–13
17. Friedman EM, de Jong AL, Sulek M (2001) Pediatric bilateral vocal fold immobility: the role of carbon dioxide laser posterior transverse partial cordectomy. Ann Otol Rhinol Laryngol 110(8):723–728
18. Preciado D, Zalzal G (2012) A systematic review of supraglottoplasty outcomes. Arch Otolaryngol Head Neck Surg 138(8):718–721
19. Zalzal GH, Anon JB, Cotton RT (1987) Epiglottoplasty for the treatment of laryngomalacia. Ann Otol Rhinol Laryngol 96(1, pt 1):72–76
20. Zalzal GH, Collins WO (2005) Microdebrider-assisted supraglottoplasty. Int J Pediatr Otorhinolaryngol 69(3):305–309.22
21. Groblewski JC, Shah RK, Zalzal GH (2009) Microdebrider-assisted supraglottoplasty for laryngomalacia. Ann Otol Rhinol Laryngol 118(8):592–597
22. Denoyelle F, Mondain M, Gresillon N, Roger G, Chaudre F, Garabedian EN (2003) Failures and complications of supraglottoplasty in children. Arch Otolaryngol Head Neck Surg 129(10):1077–1080
23. Rastatter JC, Schroeder JW, Hoff SR, Holinger LD (2010) Aspiration before and after supraglottoplasty regardless of technique. Int J Otolaryngol 2010:912814

MIX
Papier aus verantwortungsvollen Quellen
Paper from responsible sources
FSC® C105338

If you have any concerns about our products,
you can contact us on
ProductSafety@springernature.com

In case Publisher is established outside the EU,
the EU authorized representative is:
Springer Nature Customer Service Center GmbH
Europaplatz 3, 69115 Heidelberg, Germany

Printed by Libri Plureos GmbH
in Hamburg, Germany